The keys to happiness and long-term fulfilment
lie in emulating
authentic patterns of human behaviour.

With love,
SCOTT

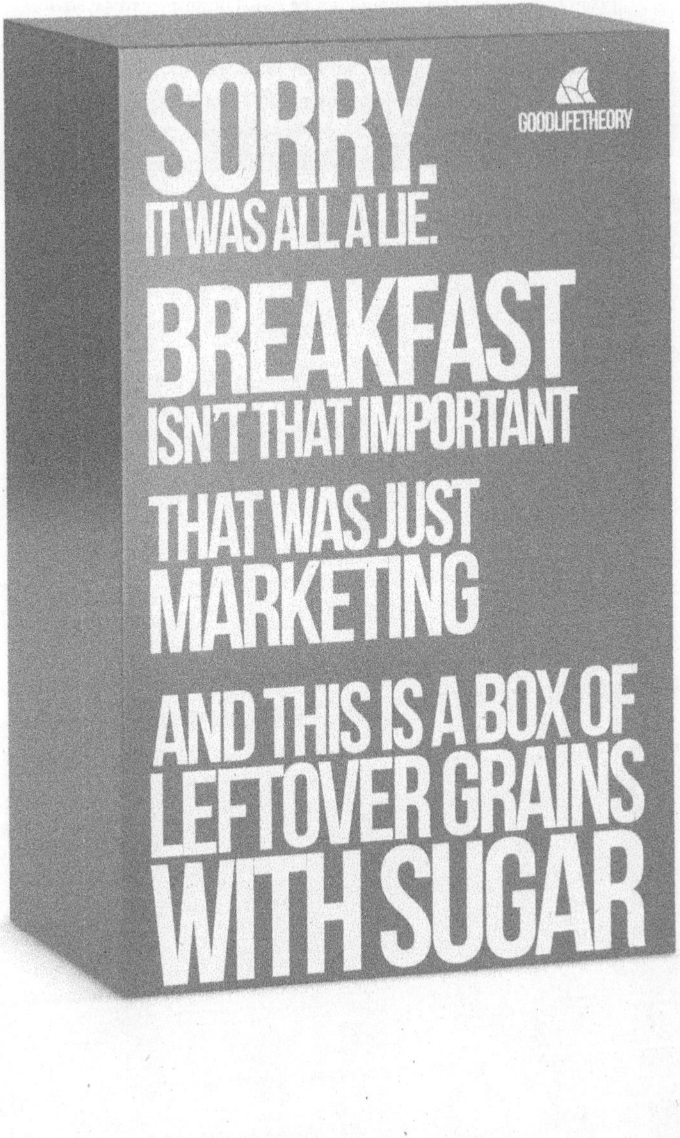
SORRY.
IT WAS ALL A LIE.
BREAKFAST
ISN'T THAT IMPORTANT
THAT WAS JUST
MARKETING
AND THIS IS A BOX OF
LEFTOVER GRAINS
WITH SUGAR
GOODLIFETHEORY

FASTING

MOTHER NATURE'S
GAME CHANGER

SCOTT MURRAY

First published in November 2019

www.goodlifetheory.com

scott@goodlifetheory.com

Copyright © Scott Murray, 2019

Printed and bound in Great Britain by Clays Ltd, Elcograf S.p.A.

A catalogue record for this book is available from the British Library

ISBN: 978-1-9162724-0-8

To everyone I have ever met
and everything that has ever happened to me.

CONTENTS

INTRODUCTION

We are constantly being shaped by seemingly irrelevant stimuli, subliminal information, and internal forces we don't know a thing about.

- ROBERT SAPOLSKY

If I told you that the last time I cried was in Copenhagen, I would be lying. The last time I cried was during a mushroom-fuelled introspective journey at a Dutch farm. But the time before that was in Copenhagen. My girlfriend at the time had just told me she wasn't in love with me anymore. Within ten minutes, I was alone and signing a form to confirm a monthly donation to a charity whose name I cannot remember. They must have seen me looking dejected and thought I was the perfect customer. At least that's the story I told myself for a while after. What I didn't mention was that in between heart-break and charitable gesture, I spent some time gazing into the eyes of a friendly labrador.

In 2015, Miho Nagasawa, a Japanese scientist at the Department of Animal Science and Biotechnology at Azabu University, discovered something that will change the way you look at dogs forever. And perhaps at life, too. He and his team found that gazing into a dog's eyes increases oxytocin release in humans. Oxytocin is the hormone responsible for love, bonding, and generosity. That friendly Danish dog had put me under a spell. And when an opportunity to be generous came along, my brain jumped at it. We think we have total agency over what we do, but the reality is much more nuanced. There are a multitude of factors influencing our decisions and behaviours that we have absolutely no idea about.

Many people like to talk about bio-hacking these days. Indeed, some have made a lot of money from it. After they throw some big words at you, they try to sell you a strange contraption or a bizarre supplement. If you ask me, it's all nonsense. The ultimate biohack is to live without expensive distractions and to emulate authentic patterns of human behaviour. Incorporating fasting is a great place to start.

Before we begin, I would like to emphasise that my desire with this project is simply to provide some information that you would not normally get through mainstream channels.
It's not something that I'm trying to sell to you. And it's not something that I'm trying to get you to believe. Because, let's face it, the world is being overrun by people standing up and telling others what they should think, what they should do, and what they should purchase. Whether its politics, science, medicine, or nutrition. They are all at it. We are constantly being told *this* is how it is. You must believe it, and if you don't believe it, well then you must be *wrong*. Conventional wisdom has been around for so long that we forget to challenge what it means. Or why we continue to repeat it. If we neglect to question common thinking, we risk sleepwalking into disaster.

All that I'm doing here is putting information before you. What you make of it is none of my business. It's your business. I'm not here to get you to believe anything, to sell you anything or to dispense medical advice. What I'm here to do is to offer the possibility that there is another way of looking at things. What I hope to do is to provide you the tools you need to empower yourself.

You are a cosmic being of infinite potential, and there is a lot you can do with what you already have.

THIS BOOK WILL BE SPLIT INTO SEVEN PARTS:

DESTRUCTIVE DIETING

*A synopsis of the principles of weight loss
and the current attitude towards dieting and fasting.*

FASTING FOR FAT LOSS

*A summary of the various ways in which fasting
can be an effective tool for fat loss.*

YOUR FASTING LIFESTYLE

A guide on how to incorporate fasting into your lifestyle.

PROLONGED FASTING

*An exploration into the properties and applications of prolonged
fasting, and what to expect.*

FASTING AND THE BRAIN

*A look into how fasting can interact with our brain
and positively impact our happiness and personal evolution.*

FASTING FOR THE FUTURE

*A discussion on how fasting can optimise health in various areas
and be used to combat several of the problems that we face today.*

FEED THE POSITIVE, STARVE THE NEGATIVE

*A collection of the most common criticisms and questions about
fasting, and my tailored responses to each one.*

Part One

DESTRUCTIVE DIETING

NO MORE DESTRUCTIVE DIETING

The real problem of humanity: we have palaeolithic emotions;
medieval institutions; and godlike technology.

- E. O. WILSON

ESDi art and design school. Barcelona. Thursday November 8, 2012. Early afternoon. I've just taken my seat for the Photoshop class. I was not aware of it, but in this hour I would receive one of the most important lessons of my short-lived educational career. It was within this hour that Fran Lopez introduced me to the concept of destructive editing.

In graphic design, destructive editing is a bad idea. It involves directly editing the original image that you are working with, meaning you cannot remove these edits if you change your mind later. There is no way back with destructive editing. And it is not a sustainable way to work. The reason this was an important lesson was not that it taught me to be a better designer. It was important because it led me to invent a similar concept: *destructive dieting*. And that's not just my dyslexia playing up.

Destructive dieting involves drastic changes and severe restriction. It searches for quick-fixes and ignores the long-term view. It takes all the elements that make us ourselves and distorts them beyond recognition. Destructive dieting is drastic, unpleasant and unsustainable. It is rather common too. But it rarely works. 80% of individuals who lose over 10% of their body weight will regain it within 12 months.

Mother Nature did not design us to diet destructively, and it is not an authentic pattern of human behaviour. She did, however, design us to look for new things, and this can be problematic. 100,000 years ago, when we roamed the African Savannah looking for food, this desire to find new things would have served us well and led to a healthy lifestyle. Today, consumer culture has exploited this hard-wired desire, leading to various destructive patterns of behaviour. Everything is *new* this, *new* that. New features. New taste. New packaging. New things fascinate us. We want the new diet. The new solution. The new way to lose weight. But we forget that the very things we need to thrive are not new. They are ancient. And we already have them. First, let's break down how we lose weight. I assure you, it's rather simple.

Some say that only hormones matter. Some say that only calories matter. But the truth lies somewhere in the middle. Rather than being black and white, it's all shades of grey. How hormones interact within the body can directly affect how many calories we consume or expend*.

Likewise, changing the amount of calories we consume or expend can also have a direct impact on our hormonal activity. Hormones and calories are not mutually exclusive. Rather, they depend on each other. So it makes little sense to disregard one or the other.

The energy balance will be the deciding factor in our weight, which is the balance between the energy we consume and the energy we expend. The amount of food we consume governs our energy intake. And the energetic requirements of our body govern the rate of energy expenditure.

---

*another word for burning calories. Think of expending as *spending* calories.

We often refer to this concept to as calories in versus calories out. I'm sure you are familiar. If we consume more calories than we burn, then we will gain weight. Likewise, if we burn more calories than we consume, we will lose weight. This makes sense for a foundation, but it falls short of useful advice. Saying that a person loses weight because they burn more calories than they consume is like saying, 'Bill Gates is wealthy because he makes more money than he spends.' I understand the concept, and I agree. I can't dispute that logic. But *how* is it that Bill Gates makes more money than he spends? *How* does he maintain it over the long term? This is where we have to consider the role that hormones and other lifestyle factors will play.

Unfortunately, many people assume that a short-term drastic diet will be an effective strategy to lose fat for good. All you have to do is restrict calories, *right?* But in reality, this is a flawed approach, and for many reasons. The main one being that the goalposts do not stay in the same place.

When we restrict calories, the body eventually adapts by reducing the rate of energy expenditure to match the new amount of energy intake. This means the body is using *less* energy, so feelings of fatigue and weakness are inevitable with destructive dieting. But it is not just the body that is using less energy. The brain has to take a hit too, which explains the prevalence of brain fog and bad moods during a destructive diet. The scientific term for this is adaptive thermogenesis, but you can think of it as the metabolism playing catch up. This may sound like an annoyance, but it is a hardwired survival mechanism. Throughout our evolution, food was never a guarantee. The body had to adapt to the food availability of the environment to ensure survival, and it has meant that you and I are able to complain about it today. However, our modern food environment is not changing often, so this adaptive mechanism is not so useful. That the metabolism can adapt helps to explain why people quickly rebound from periods of highly restrictive dieting and revert to more or less their original weight. If you stop eating ice cream for two months, what will happen when you start again? Your body will adapt, and you will gain weight. When we subscribe to destructive diets and drastically restrict our calories, the body has no choice but to adapt. It won't happen immediately, but it will happen. This is problematic precisely because diets have a time limit. When you finish the diet, what happens? You go back to your lifestyle and the body will do what it does best: *adapt*.

Destructive dieting comes with a price. Resorting to drastic measures to lose weight is like taking out a loan with absurd conditions; there will *always* be interest to pay later on. No one gets rich from taking out Payday loans. And no one achieves sustainable fat loss with destructive dieting. The body is intelligent, resilient, and constantly adapting. We cannot work against it; we must work with it.

Destructive diets will not work.

We have to think of lifestyles and the long game. We need to emulate authentic patterns of human behaviour.

It's time to step outside the box.

A NEW PERSPECTIVE

Conformity is the jailer of freedom and the enemy of growth.

- JOHN F. KENNEDY

To better explain fasting, I will have to introduce two characters that will make several appearances throughout this book: Zug and Mo.

Zug lives in prehistoric times, whereas Mo lives in the year 2019. Zug is a hunter-gatherer who has to find his own food. And usually goes from anywhere between 16 to 24 hours between his last meal of the day and his first the following day. Sometimes he will go even longer than 24 hours between meals, but rarely less. Zug is no stranger to periods of food scarcity and has gone several days eating nothing before. The longest period that Mo has between his last meal of the day and his breakfast is about eight hours. And that is because he's in bed. Mainstream media bombards him with propaganda claiming that breakfast is the most important meal of the day and he must eat frequently to be healthy. Mo's longest period without food was about half a day. And he never stopped complaining about it. Zug spends most of the day on the move. Mo spends most of the day sitting on his arse.

Although there are many years between Zug and Mo, it is only a blink of the eye in evolutionary terms. Our genetic coding has remained the same, yet our attitude towards fasting has changed drastically. How did this happen?

The first thing to consider is that, as humans, we like to fit in with the group. We are all conditioned to want approval from others. It was important for our evolution as a social species, and it served us well in the past. But it is important that we do not let it own us now. Life is like a game of Tetris. If you try to fit in, you will disappear. Conformity is one of the few authentic patterns of human behaviour that I would *not* suggest emulating.

In the 1950s, psychologist Solomon Asch explored the concept of conformity. In his experiments, he showed student volunteers a picture of three lines that varied in length. He then asked them questions about the picture, such as which line was the longest. The questions were so simple that 95 percent of the participants got the correct answer to every question. But things got a little spicy when Asch added some confederates into the mix. In psychology, confederates are actors who take part in the experiment, pretending to be a participant but in actuality working for the researcher. Here, the aim of the confederates was to influence the answer of the naïve participants and pressure them into conforming. They would do this by giving incorrect answers to these simple questions. When the actors became the majority in the group and gave the same incorrect answer, the number of participants who gave correct answers to all the questions dropped from 95 percent to 25 percent. That means 75 percent of participants went along with the wrong answer just because most people in the room were saying it. This tells us we are susceptible to conform, but it does not tell us exactly *why*. Were the participants scared of being the odd one out? Or had peer pressure altered their actual perception of reality? Fifty-five years on from Asch's original study, neuroscientist Gregory Berns may have an answer.

Berns and his team from Emory University recruited thirty-two volunteers and had them play a game. They showed each participant two different three-dimensional objects on a computer screen and asked them to decide whether they could rotate the first object to match the second. In one condition, the participants played on their own. In another, they played in a group in which most participants were actors who would give the same wrong answers, much like in Asch's experiment. The researchers used fMRI scans* to observe activity in the brains of participants as they played the game in both of these conditions. The results were interesting. But a little disturbing too, as you will see.

When the participants played alone, they gave the wrong answer 13.8 percent of the time. When they played in a group with actors who were deliberately answering incorrectly, they gave the wrong answers 41 percent of the time. After learning about Asch's experiments, we could predict this would happen. But Bern's study revealed some additional insight why. When the volunteers played alone, the brain scans showed activity in a network of brain regions including the occipital cortex and parietal cortex, which we associate with visual and spatial perception. Playing the game alone also heightened activity in the frontal cortex, which is responsible for conscious decision-making. But when the participants played in a group, and conformed to the wrong answer of the majority, their brain activity revealed something different. Remember, what we want to know is whether people conform despite knowing that the group is wrong, or whether the influence of the group alters their perception of reality.

If people know that they are giving a wrong answer to fit in with the group, then we should see more brain activity in the decision-making prefrontal cortex. However, if the brain scans showed heightened activity in regions associated with visual and spatial perception, it would suggest that the group influence had changed the participants' perception of reality. And that was exactly what happened. The participants who conformed to the mistaken majority showed less brain activity in the frontal, decision-making regions, and more in the areas associated with perception. They were approaching the problem

*fMRI stands for functional magnetic resonance imaging machine, which can measure which parts of the brain are active when you're thinking a particular thought or performing a specific task.

differently. And totally unaware that the group influence was making them do it. People often say that peer pressure is unpleasant. And that is true. But what they don't say is that it can change your actual perception of the world. And that is even more worrying.

The opinion of the group is a powerful mind-altering substance. If the group thinks breakfast is the most important meal of the day, then you are more likely to believe that too. It's not a case of agreeing with the majority because you are unsure, or trying to save face and fit in. Oh no. What is happening is much more extraordinary. And very dangerous. When the group believes something, your perceptions of reality can change to match this belief. In the study we just mentioned, most of the participants said that they agreed with the group because 'they thought they had arrived serendipitously at the same correct answer'. The participants had no idea that the group had influenced them. But it had, in a big way. They thought they were giving the right answer, even though it was the wrong one, and probably not one they would have chosen had they been on their own. When you understand this phenomenon, you can see it all throughout history and in modern society. We are prone to conform. And to make matters worse, our biological design does not like standing out.

At this stage, you might think *but not all the participants in these studies conformed*. And you would be right. A few of them still picked the answer they knew to be right despite the group influence. And the resulting brain scans revealed a lot about the psychology of standing out. When participants went against the group, it heightened activation in the amygdala, a region in the brain associated with upsetting emotions such as the fear of rejection*. Gregory Berns refers to this as the 'pain of independence'. The group influence can literally change our perceptions. And going against the majority can activate primitive, powerful and unconscious feelings of rejection, fear, and

---

*It is also a region we will cover in more detail in chapter five.

anxiety. Standing out is difficult. It is much easier to conform. Going against the group takes courage, and your brain does not want you to do it. But sometimes, we have to do it.

Our perceptions make reality. And the consensus of the group influences our perceptions. For years, most people have said things like *fasting is unhealthy, breakfast is the most important meal of the day* and *we must eat frequently*. These mantras have been repeated so often and by such a large majority that people genuinely believe them. This is their *perception* of reality, but it is not *reality*. Going against what the group thinks is hard, but I'm here to help.

To discover the second reason as to why fasting has been forgotten, you just have to think about who will profit from fasting.

That's right. *No one.* No multi-million dollar supplement companies. No snack giants. No fad diet peddlers. Fasting is for the people. And it always will be. But don't get your tin foil hat out just yet, because there is a little more to it. Perhaps it's not all so sinister.

Since I was a wee boy, people have been saying that eating small meals as frequently as possible is healthy. They have also told me many times that breakfast is the most important meal of the day and that skipping it is unhealthy. How did this happen?

First, the mantra of *breakfast is the most important meal of the day* is a nonsense created by the Kellogg propaganda machine. It is a claim that to this day lacks any credible evidence. But we debunk that myth in chapter six. Convincing people that they must eat frequently will line the pockets of many greedy companies. But again, perhaps it is not all so sinister.

Not so long ago, the overwhelming perception was that eating frequent small meals would speed up the metabolism, and lead to fat loss. This was advice the nutritional establishment, doctors and mainstream media repeated with pride. But it makes no sense, and it is awful advice for anyone looking to lose fat or get healthy. How did we ever believe that eating *more* would lead to weight loss? And who has the time to be preparing and eating meals all throughout the day? It's ridiculous. But there may be an inkling of science behind it.

The idea that eating frequently will speed up your metabolism comes from the thermic effect of food. This is the amount of energy that your body will use to digest food. In theory, eating frequently *will* speed up your metabolism. If you eat more, then you will expend more energy throughout the day, as the body has to spend energy to process and digest the food. To appear science-based, people took this idea and concluded that eating frequently was the key to weight loss, because it would increase energy expenditure and make the energy balance easier to manage. But hold on a second. This makes little sense either. Allow me to explain why.

First, if someone is spending more time eating, then they will do fewer activities that require more energy. And no one feels active right after they have eaten, so a period of natural inactivity will follow each meal. If someone is busy preparing, eating, and digesting meals, they are not spending that time being active. And the energy we spend on digesting food pales in comparison to the energy we spend being active. For example, if you eat just one meal a day but stay active for the rest of the time, you will burn a lot more energy than if you spend the day trying to eat as frequently as possible.

Second, the increase in energy expenditure from eating is so slight and short-lived that the only way to make it count regarding weight loss would be to eat *all the time*. From the moment you wake until the moment you go to sleep. Now, you need not be a scientist to work out that if someone is eating all the time, they will not be losing weight. Unless perhaps they are only allowing themselves to eat celery or something similar, which is not an approach that I imagine being too pleasant or sustainable.

The idea that we should eat frequently is nonsense, and it may have even done more damage than the nutritional establishment would care to admit. Acting on this advice will not bring any positive results, and it may even leave a person in worse shape than before they started. And besides, this is not to mention the simple fact that small meals are not satisfying nor enjoyable. Small, unsatisfying meals make you want to eat *more*, not less. I also recall being told that eating small meals throughout the day would help to control my hunger. But this is also nonsense. Who has ever had their hunger go away after eating a small meal? The opposite happens. Eating a small meal opens the floodgates of hunger. That's why we have starters and appetisers.

I do not know how we ever fell for any of this nonsense. But we can see through it now. Do you believe that Mother Nature designed human beings to graze on small meals? Does anyone believe that?

If you consider that for most of our time on earth we did not have a consistent food supply and could only eat sporadically, it makes no sense. Remember, they only invented home fridges in 1913. Eating frequently is born out of modern design. It is not an authentic pattern of human behaviour. Big, satisfying meals are what we crave, and ironically, they may also be integral to losing fat and keeping it off. All of this so-called advice from the so-called professionals seems to have taken us backwards. Society is not hunter-gatherer anymore, but our genetic design is. So we would be foolish to ignore these authentic patterns of human behaviour from a health perspective.

It's time to take back control and change the game. One of the most beneficial things we can do regarding *when* we eat is something we've been doing for a long time. Zug and his hominid friends did it, the Ancient Greeks and Egyptians did it, several religions continue to do it and many people are waking up and starting to do it now. It's free, it's easy, it enhances the enjoyment of food and it will simplify your life.

It's fasting.

INTRODUCING THE GAME CHANGER

Innovation happens when you change the game; you bring a different twist to what is currently established and perceived.

- PEARL ZHU

Fasting* is the voluntary abstinence from food. Despite what many people claim, fasting is not the same as starvation. By definition, they are opposites. Fasting is a choice. Starving is not.

Once roughly twelve hours have passed since our last meal, we enter the postabsorptive state, also known as the fasted state. This is where the body has depleted the energy from food and turns its attention inward to break down stored fat for fuel. Contrary to popular belief, you will not shrivel up and die after twelve hours without food. In fact, you may even feel full of life. You have just unlocked a whole new energy source. But more on that shortly.

Fasting is not new, but it *is* enjoying a renaissance. There are two reasons why. The first is that people are waking up. And the second is the information coming out. Emerging research continues to suggest that fasting could have therapeutic potential in combatting the pandemics of obesity and type 2 diabetes.

There are many benefits to fasting. But we can't fast forever, or we would die.

---

*To clarify, when I talk about fasting in this book, I am referring to water fasting, in which drinking water during the fast is essential and encouraged.

Therefore, we must cycle periods of fasting with periods of feeding, and this is where the *intermittent* part comes in.

Intermittent fasting involves taking the twenty-four hours of the day and splitting it up into two parts: the fasting window and the feeding window. To enter the fasted state, the fasting window should be at least twelve hours, but remember that this will also include the time that you spend sleeping. Don't worry too much about the specifics of the timeframe just yet. The beauty of fasting lies in the flexible nature and how it can simplify life, and we will cover it all in great depth during part three.

There are other methods to incorporate fasting, such as alternate day fasting or the 5:2 method, but I recommend the intermittent approach and splitting each day into fasting and feeding. Arguably, this is the most sustainable approach. But as long as fasting is being used to benefit your life, it is not all that important how you do it.

Many people, when they hear of intermittent fasting, are quick to assume that they are already doing it. The vast majority of them are mistaken. Many think that fasting is just refraining from eating in the conventional sense of consuming a solid meal. But it is the abstinence from *all* calorie consumption, whether those calories come from liquids, meals, snacks, or anything in between.

Some people do not have time for a proper breakfast, so they will instead opt for some kind of shake or smoothie. Although it may not *feel* like eating in the traditional sense, these items still contain a significant amount of calories. Some people skip breakfast altogether and go for a coffee with milk and sugar, or perhaps a calorific syrup-laden brew available in all big coffee chains. It may *feel* like skipping breakfast because they are not eating a meal, but they are still consuming calories. Some people finish dinner early, but then drink wine until late. Unfortunately, all alcoholic drinks, including wine, contain calories. In reality, most people are nowhere near fasting.

Energy comes from many sources. If we are consuming energy, we are feeding the body. Not fasting. For many people, the only time in which they allow their digestive system a break from all that work is when they are sleeping.

In 2015, renowned fasting researcher Dr. Satchin Panda and his team at the Salk Institute of Biological Studies created an app that allowed participants to track the timing of their calorie consumption. The researchers monitored the participants for three weeks to see if there were any patterns regarding the timing of their eating behaviour. They found that the average time span from the moment the participants began to consume calories until they finished for the day was fourteen hours and forty-five minutes. If we are to assume that the participants were sleeping for eight hours a night, this means they would have been consuming calories for almost the entire day. In fact, only 9.7% of the participants had a daily eating duration of fewer than twelve hours. This was only the first part of the study. For the next sixteen weeks, the researchers asked the participants to restrict the timeframe of their calorie consumption to just ten hours a day. The results were fascinating. Although they did not ask the participants to change the amount they ate, they consumed fewer calories overall because of this time restriction on eating, leading to fat loss. They also reported having better quality sleep, less hunger, and more energy. In fact, the participants enjoyed the time-restricted eating schedule so much that they all voluntarily carried on with it even after the study had finished. Dr. Panda checked in with the participants thirty-six weeks after the study had finished. What do you think happened? All of them had maintained their weight loss, while their sleep and energy levels continued to improve. They adjusted *when* they ate, and the rest took care of itself.

In 2018, researchers from the University of Illinois wanted to investigate what impact intermittent fasting could have on the body weight of obese adults. They assigned participants to a fasting group, in which they would fast for sixteen hours of the day and eat for eight. The researchers allowed participants to eat as much as they desired during these eight hours. There were no restrictions on what they could eat, nor were they required to monitor their calorie intake. By the end of the twelve week study period, the participants were still losing fat, even though they were eating as much as they liked. Without even trying, they restricted their calorie intake with fasting and lost fat. They didn't have to do anything destructive. Intermittent fasting made losing fat *effortless* for them. Their blood pressure even decreased too, so this method of fat loss could not have been very stressful.

They adjusted *when* they ate, and the rest took care of itself.

Fasting will change the game of fat loss. Let's explore why.

Part Two

FASTING FOR FAT LOSS

In the game of destructive dieting, there is no winner.

Fasting is an authentic pattern of human behaviour,
and embracing it will allow us to thrive in the third millennium.

Incorporating fasting into your lifestyle
will enhance the enjoyment of food and of everyday life.

In this section, we will cover how fasting makes fat loss effortless.

METABOLIC FLEXIBILITY, FAT BURNING, AND TERRY

The human capacity for burden is like bamboo- far more flexible than you'd ever believe at first glance.

- JODI PICOULT

Macronutrients and micronutrients make up the food we eat. Macronutrients are protein, fats, and carbohydrates, whereas micronutrients are things like vitamins and minerals. How the digestive system responds to the food we eat depends on the macronutrient profile. We break dietary protein down into amino acids, which are the building blocks of proteins* responsible for the maintenance and growth of muscle, skin and connective tissue. We convert fat into fatty acids, which are vital to human life. They help the proteins do their job while regulating our growth, immune system and reproductive health. We break carbohydrates down into glucose, which the body and brain can use as a source of energy.

When we eat, our blood sugar levels rise. This means we have the energy source of glucose in our bloodstream. But it cannot access the cells alone. To access the cells and deliver the energy, we need insulin. Produced by the pancreas, insulin is an anabolic hormone that helps with the uptake of amino acids and proteins, which are essential for

---

* Proteins are large, complex molecules that play many critical roles in the body. They do most of the work in cells and are required for the structure, function, and regulation of the body's tissues and organs.

growth. It is also responsible for storing any excess energy that we consume as body fat. The main responsibility of insulin is to control levels of glucose in the blood and process the uptake of energy and nutrients.

When we eat, glucose enters the bloodstream and insulin rises to take the glucose out of the blood and shuttle it into the cells around the brain and body. Insulin is the key that opens the cell and allows energy to enter. It allows us to break down the food we consume and use it as energy. Once we have met the immediate energetic requirements of the body, we must then store any excess energy for later. Remember, we have evolved with periods of food scarcity, so being able to store energy from food for later use is a necessity in our story of survival. Excess energy is first stored in the liver and muscles as glycogen, which is a storage form of glucose that we can use for energy whenever the body requires it. If we have consumed enough energy to fill the glycogen reserves, we then convert it into fatty acids via a process called de novo lipogenesis. This literally means 'to make new fat' and we do this so we can transport the energy for storage in the fat cells. We can then break this stored fat down for energy whenever we face a period of food scarcity. But this presents us with a problem. We don't face periods of food scarcity anymore. Eating frequently is a recent development in human history. If we consult the numbers, we see a strong correlation between the popularity of eating frequently and the rapid rise in obesity. This does not mean that the recent development of eating often is the root cause of obesity, but it is not helping the situation. Allowing the body to burn off some stored energy can only be beneficial. And to do that, we need to emulate authentic patterns of human behaviour. More on that in a moment.

When you eat more than you need, you give the body no choice but to store the excess as body fat. It's similar to payday. First, you pay off all the urgent costs like the electricity bill, which acts as the immediate energy needs of the body. Then, you withdraw some cash to have on hand just in case. This cash represents the glycogen reserves. If there is anything left over, you deposit it into the bank of body fat, which you can access when times get tough.

Let's be clear, we are not fat. Rather, we *have* fat, and we can use this fat for energy. If we want to lose body fat, then we need to give our body a reason to do so. And encouraging the body to use it as fuel would be a compelling one. Body fat has a purpose. And a rather profound one at that. It is not a punishment, and it does not define who you are. Fat does not have to be a source of self-loathing. In fact, you can use it for something very useful: *energy*.

Today, most of the human population has easy access to food. But in terms of our evolutionary history, this is a recent development. Throughout the ages, humans had to rely on hunting and gathering food with their own hands. Therefore, we have evolved with regular periods of food scarcity. According to our DNA, eating was never a guarantee, so Mother Nature has prepared us for food scarcity.

If humans could not withstand periods of food scarcity, then you and I would not be here today. Evolution has imprinted fasting into our DNA.

You may resent fat storage, but it helped us evolve, providing us with an alternative fuel source for when times get tough. However, like I said, times don't get tough anymore, and this can throw a spanner into the works. Our system for storing fat works well when we are operating in the environment we evolved in. Today, hyper-palatable and calorie-dense foods that cause a spasm in dopamine and that are available at every corner have hijacked this system.

Some say that controlling insulin is an effective strategy to lose body fat. When insulin is low, the body can tap into stored fat and utilise it for energy. If we are not eating anything, it is impossible to raise insulin, so the body looks inwards and starts breaking down fat for fuel. We call this process lipolysis, and it produces ketone bodies, which are an energy source for the body and the brain. Some people say that controlling insulin is the *only* way to lose fat, but this is a flawed approach. Breaking down and burning stored fat for energy is not the same as losing body fat for good. Fat-burn does not always equate to fat-loss. During a period of fasting, you can deplete glucose and glycogen stores, lower insulin, and break down stored body fat for fuel. But if you proceed to consume more energy than your body requires during the subsequent feeding period, you will store this excess energy as body fat. And you are back at square one. We cannot sidestep the fundamental principles. Controlling insulin is just one part of the equation; we still need to be mindful of our calorie intake and consider the big picture. With that said, controlling insulin can be a good target to aim for, as it will usually lead to a healthier lifestyle. We do not have magical solutions, but we do have many tools available. And it is much easier to do an excellent job if you equip yourself with an expansive toolbox as opposed to a limited one. The mission is clear: expand the toolbox. And becoming more metabolically flexible is a great way to do so.

Metabolic flexibility is the ability to switch between the two fuel sources of glucose and fat. Researchers have linked metabolic inflexibility to physical inactivity, overeating, and obesity. Relying on one fuel source and neglecting the other makes fat loss a struggle. Let's explore why this might be.

A few years ago, Mo's go-to breakfast was a bowl of cereal and a few slices of toast. Conventional wisdom had convinced him that this kind of meal would give him energy for the whole day, but he was falling asleep before lunch. In reality, Mo was not setting himself up for an energetic day. Rather, he was committing what I like to call *carbicide*. Mo thought such a breakfast would keep him full, but within hours ravenous hunger would consume him. This was not an ideal situation, but Mo thought it was a natural part of life. He never stopped to consider that he was living unnaturally. The thought he might be metabolically inflexible never crossed his mind. In those days, Mo was over reliant on using glucose for fuel, which is why his body would panic with hunger and tiredness whenever it started to run low. He never allowed his body to follow the natural rhythm of depleting glucose and burning fat. In fact, his body probably did not understand that it *could* burn fat for fuel. Like so many others, he was a slave to glucose and eating frequently. Fortunately, he found a way out.

After around twelve hours of fasting, the body has now more or less depleted glucose and has to think about metabolising an alternative fuel source to survive. To do so, it has to exercise flexibility. The body may not be familiar with this process, which is why fasting can be a little uncomfortable at first for some people, but it will adapt. We do not have to eat all the time. Big companies that sell snacks and meal replacements wish we did. But we don't. When you grasp this concept, the game will change. You don't *have* to suffer that dreaded pre-lunchtime crash. You don't *have* to worry about when, where and what to eat at all hours of the day. You don't *have* to eat breakfast. You don't *have* to be a slave to hunger. You can fast. And you can *thrive*. Metabolic flexibility is a useful tool that you can use to engineer sustainable fat loss. To gain it, all you need to do is emulate authentic patterns of human behaviour. All you need to do is *fast*. Eating frequently is an obsolete system that has enslaved many. When you take yourself out of this system, you will see how flawed it is.

Metabolic flexibility comes with stable energy levels. The mid-morning crash that Mo used to suffer is a common phenomenon in offices all over the world, and it is largely a result of being reliant on glucose. However, it does not have to be like this. When the body can transition between fuel sources, there is no need to panic when glucose runs low. If you are metabolically flexible and glucose becomes depleted, then it's okay, you can burn fat for fuel instead. Without the crash, your energy levels remains stable over the course of the day. Consider Zug. During a period of food scarcity, Zug needs consistent energy levels to find food and stay alive. If humans could not maintain consistent energy levels during periods of fasting, then we would not have survived until today. Fasting, and burning fat for fuel, keeps your energy levels consistent. If we consult the research we see that those who burn more fat for fuel (or have higher rates of *fat oxidation*, to be scientific) are more successful in maintaining their weight loss. In fact, scientists agree that *lower* rates of fat oxidation are strong predictors of weight gain and obesity. Incorporating fasting teaches us to burn fat for fuel, which makes fat loss easier, and stops it from coming back.

Destructive dieting approaches have an end date. Afterwards, people will regain most, or all, of the weight than they had originally lost. This is because they return to their normal lifestyle, and the body adapts. Maybe you have seen this happen before or even experienced it yourself. To explain it in more detail, let's take Terry from down the road.

After waking up with a raging hangover following an evening of beer and curry, Terry decides that he will go on a diet. He puts a few months of no booze, excessive cardio, and eating only chicken and broccoli in the calendar. Unsurprisingly, he loses a significant amount of weight. Terry celebrates by going out for a curry with extra naan and several pints of lager. Although he maintains some healthy habits that he picked up from his diet, he reverts to his normal lifestyle of curry and booze. It's not long before Terry's body catches up, and he's back to the weight he was before he started his diet. Our mate Terry didn't consider the long-term view. Don't be like Terry.

Fat loss is simple. It's not easy, but it *is* simple. Keeping the fat off for good, however, can be challenging. The biggest problem with the popular concept of diets is that they neglect the long-term view, and this makes them destructive. Anyone can go on a strict diet for two months, but what happens afterwards? What is the point of punishing yourself only to return to square one soon after? We must focus on sustainability, and therefore it's all about the lifestyle. Dieting, in the conventional sense of having a start and end point to a period of restriction, is nonsense. It is a flawed method, and I do not know why we persist with it. We must think about the lifestyle. It may not deliver such swift results in the short-term, but the long-term developments will be infinitely more valuable.

People like Terry all over the world are struggling with destructive dieting. Perhaps they decided one day to go hard on the diet. They gave up several things they enjoyed, went running for hours on end, restricted their calorie intake drastically and ended up losing a lot of weight. Feeling miserable, yes, but losing weight. There was a target to reach. Perhaps they had a goal weight in mind or a finish date. So what happens when they reach said target? They will go back to the way they were living before. And just like with Terry from down the road, the weight will come right back with even more vigour than before. This happens time and time again, but people still do not see it. The problem is not the start; it is the end.

People like Terry don't prepare for life after the diet, and so it all goes pear-shaped.

Forget the diet.

Forget punishing yourself.

It's time to turn this upside down. You do not need a diet. You need a lifestyle that allows for vacations, social commitments, and *living*. Incorporating fasting is a great place to start, and metabolic flexibility is one aspect as to why.

But let's explore more.

APPETITE CONTROL, GREMLINS, AND THE TRUTH ABOUT HUNGER

Hunger is the first element of self-discipline. If you can control what you eat and drink, you can control everything else.

- SHAYKH DR. UMAR FARUQ ABD-ALLAH

Hunger is real. But it is not at all what you think it is. Let me explain.

Although leptin and ghrelin sound like goblin warlords, they are in fact the hunger hormones. Leptin is responsible for satiety. It lets you know that it is time to stop eating by sending a satisfaction signal to the brain. Ghrelin does the opposite. It increases your appetite and lets you know that it is time to eat.

After its discovery in 1994, many companies invested large sums of money to attain the rights of leptin. They did so on the assumption that they could create a medication that would not only reverse obesity but also make them a huge profit in doing so. If leptin suppresses appetite and is responsible for the satisfaction signal, the cure for obesity must be to increase leptin. Sounds straightforward so far. Indeed, it would be a settlement that benefitted both parties. A true win-win situation. But reality is not always so simple. The plan fell through when researchers found that obese people already had high levels of leptin, so giving them more would not be the answer. In obesity, there is *too much* leptin. Not too little. But if leptin is high in obesity, then surely their appetite would be non-existent, and it would only be a matter of time before they lose weight? The situation is puzzling. To shed some light on it, let's take a deep dive on leptin.

Fat cells produce leptin. The more fat we have, the more leptin we produce. Increasing leptin as we store more fat is an evolutionary survival mechanism. Storing a certain amount of fat is beneficial to our survival, as it provides a fuel source when food is scarce. However, storing too much has the opposite effect. It makes us heavier, slower, and more appetising to predators. Mother Nature had to establish the balance of fat storage. And leptin helped her to achieve this. But recently, something has upset the balance. And as you may have guessed, the modern lifestyle is to blame. Straying from authentic patterns of human behaviour has caused the leptin system to malfunction.

Leptin makes us feel satisfied. But producing too much too quickly over a long period results in leptin *resistance*. Chronically elevated levels of leptin flood the system, preventing the satisfaction signal from reaching the brain. Have you ever met someone who is overweight yet always hungry? After finishing a meal, they still have room for more. This shows leptin struggling to do its job. When leptin becomes less effective, the brain does not receive the satisfaction signal, leaving the individual with an appetite that never goes away. In cases like this, the brain is being tricked. And the unnatural way of living is to blame. With modern food availability, we now have the means to gain body fat at a rapid rate, which ambushes the leptin feedback system and renders it useless. In leptin resistance, the lack of a satisfaction signal convinces the brain the body is starving. But in reality, the body has more stored fat than it could ever need.

We often blame an inability to lose weight or to eat less on a lack of willpower. But the situation is usually more complicated. And for someone with leptin resistance, it is hard to take control. Mother Nature designed the leptin system with a simpler time in mind. This modern lifestyle that we live, with calorie-dense and hyper-palatable foods available in abundance, can be problematic for the leptin system. To get leptin back to its best, we must reconnect with our evolutionary design.

To reverse leptin resistance, we need *sensitivity*. And to increase leptin sensitivity, we need regular periods of low leptin. This is where fasting can help. Obviously, we are not eating when we fast, so there is not yet any need to send the satisfaction signal. Therefore, leptin remains low and sensitivity increases, so when we eat, the signal is stronger. Many people find less food than usual satisfies them with a fasting lifestyle, because they have become more sensitive to leptin. Fasting helps to sensitize us to the satiating effect of Leptin and stops us going back for seconds. Think of it as Mother Nature's very own form of portion control. Often, when people fast, they expect their appetite will be impossible to satisfy when they break the fast. But the opposite happens. They thought they would eat everything in sight, but end up feeling satisfied with a modest meal. This has been the case for me, and it's a clear example of becoming more sensitive to the leptin signal of satisfaction.

Many people see hunger as a *debt* that accumulates the longer we do not eat. For example, the longer that a person fasts for, the more they will eat, which makes the whole process rather pointless. However, this idea only makes sense if we limit ourselves to the old way of thinking.

Alex Johnstone, a professor of nutrition at the University of Aberdeen, explored this concept in more detail. Her and her team at the Rowett Institute took twenty-four participants and assigned them to one of two groups. In the first group, participants would fast for thirty-six hours and could then eat as much as they liked. The fast ended at 8 am on the last day of the study, so they had an entire day to eat. In the second group, participants would eat as normal until this last day, in which they could also eat as much as they liked. Therefore, the researchers could directly compare the eating habits of people who had fasted for thirty-six hours and people who had not fasted at all. What do you think happened?

When asked this question, most people assume that the fasting group will lose control and eat a huge amount. But the results paint a different picture.

Participants who were fasting ate more, but only at breakfast. Afterwards, they reported similar hunger levels and recorded similar eating patterns to the other group throughout the day. By the end of the day, those who had fasted before only ate slightly more than those who did not. And if we consider that the fast itself had created a calorie deficit of around 2800 calories, then the implications for fat loss and tackling obesity could be huge. Professor Johnstone concluded: 'These data suggest that a 36 hour fast did not induce a powerful, unconditioned stimulus to compensate on the subsequent day.' Fasting does not create a hunger debt. And despite what many think, appetite will be easy to control. Even when coming off a fast as long as thirty-six hours.

Fasting increases leptin sensitivity, which is a powerful tool in not only losing fat but also keeping it off. Sensitivity to leptin and the satisfaction signal is Mother Nature's way of regulating our appetite and keeping us at a healthy weight. A fasting lifestyle also allows for bigger meals, which will *always* be more satisfying than smaller meals. Let's say I have 2500 calories' worth of food that I'm planning to eat in one day. If I have to divide this up and ration it throughout the day, I'll end up with a smattering of small meals that will never satisfy my hunger. However, if I was to condense this 2500 calories into a small window of time, or even just one meal, then the dining experience will be significantly more satisfying. Evolution did not design us to be happy with small meals. Big meals are where it's at.

Leptin is responsible for satiety. Ghrelin is responsible for hunger.

Leptin signals when it's time to stop eating. Ghrelin signals when it's time to *start*. Ghrelin's job is to protect us from starvation and losing too much body fat. That sounds strange, as losing fat is rarely easy in the modern world. But throughout most of our evolution, food was scarce. Losing fat causes ghrelin levels to increase as a defence mechanism. Obesity researcher David Cummings and his team at the University of Washington found that dieting for six months increased ghrelin by 24% in obese subjects. One case study from the Fitchburg State University in Massachusetts followed the journey of a natural bodybuilder preparing for a physique competition. Six months of intense dieting to reach a low body fat percentage raised ghrelin by 40%. His appetite was almost double from when he started the diet.

The brain views stored fat as energy we can use in emergency situations like food scarcity. Because of this, when we diet destructively and rapidly lose body fat, ghrelin reacts to stop it from happening. And it does this by increasing hunger. Of course, we know that losing body fat in this day and age does not pose any significant threat to our survival. Food is everywhere, and we can easily prepare a feast in a matter of minutes without risking attack by sabre-toothed tigers. However, we did not evolve with such luxuries. So stimulating hunger is what the brain does in response to losing body fat.

This explains one reason destructive dieting is so hard, and only gets harder. As you continue to lose fat with destructive methods, the brain activates various defence mechanisms to stop it from happening. Increasing ghrelin to stimulate appetite is one of these mechanisms. Managing ghrelin and keeping our appetite under control will be key in creating a healthy lifestyle. So how do we do it?

One method is to sleep more. But we will talk about that later. For now, let's focus on fasting.

In 2005, Giancarlo Natalucci and his team at the University of Vienna wanted to see what impact fasting would have on ghrelin.

They asked participants to fast for twenty-four-hours and monitored levels of ghrelin throughout. The results were not at all what they anticipated.

During the twenty-four-hour fast, ghrelin did not accumulate the longer the participants went without eating. Rather, it spiked at the familiar meal times of breakfast, lunch, and dinner. And came back down shortly afterwards. Levels of ghrelin returned to baseline even though the participants ate nothing. This tells us that hunger is like a *wave*. It crashes down, sticks around for a bit, and then goes away. Even if you eat nothing. If you are already used to fasting, you will have experienced this for yourself. Hunger does not last. It comes in a wave. And if you dive into it and wait half an hour, it subsides into a calm and content appetite. Interestingly, Doctor Natalucci also noted that 'an overall decrease in ghrelin levels was observed during the study period', signifying that fasting did not stimulate appetite. In fact, it had quite the opposite effect. Hunger comes in waves, and these waves become less powerful as the fast goes on. These are fascinating findings, and good news for anyone worried that fasting will send their appetite out of control. But what are these results *really* telling us?

They are telling us that hunger is nothing like we think it is. Conventional wisdom insists that hunger is a biological requirement for food. But perhaps it's just a brain signal. Emerging research from the Harvard Medical School suggests that the spikes in ghrelin are more closely linked to our internal circadian clock as opposed to actual food intake. In other words, hunger is a conditioned behaviour. But I will go one step further and say that these hunger waves are motivational cues to find food. Think about it. For the vast majority of our time on earth, we lived as hunter-gatherers and had to find food with our own hands. The food availability and abundance that we enjoy today only represents an evolutionary millisecond. Today, we have food everywhere. When this hunger hits, we can eat immediately. But this is not what Mother Nature designed it for. Hunger is a brain signal that motivates us to get out there and find food.

Zug is sitting in a dark cave. It's cold, it's wet, and going outside to bear the elements and find food does not seem like the most enticing prospect. Zug is more than content to stay inside in safety. But then, his stomach rumbles. Ghrelin hits. And it reminds Zug why he needs to get out there and find food. Hunger is the motivating factor that gets Zug out of the cave and on the hunt for food. For many years, we *needed* hunger to motivate us when times were hard. It has been a fundamental factor in the story of human survival.

These hunger cues are still part of our design, but we find ourselves in an environment where food is abundant. This has led to many people eating all the time. And the results are not great, with obesity rates rapidly rising. We consider this normal. But it is *abnormal* behaviour. We must question the conventional wisdom, or we risk sleepwalking into disaster.

It makes matters more complicated when some doctors and many nutritionists oppose the act of ignoring hunger. They say you should just listen to your body and eat when you're hungry. Not even that, there are people dispensing this worthless advice and having the nerve to charge money for it. They do not understand what hunger is, yet they advise we entertain it every time it strikes. Hunger is not always a biological requirement for energy. It is a brain signal that kept us alive for all those years when food was scarce.

Whatever the case may be, more and more studies show that a fasting lifestyle reduces appetite. Conventional wisdom insists that hunger will be problematic during periods of fasting. But fasting makes it *easier* to manage hunger.

I would even say that fasting is Mother Nature's most potent appetite suppressant.

FASTED ENERGY, TIDY FAT LOSS, AND MOTHER NATURE'S PEP TALK

The most durable results happen as a series of good decisions that accumulate one upon another over a very long period of time.

- SHANE PARRISH

Those who use destructive dieting bemoan a lack of energy.

With fasting in your life, you will feel more like a Patagonian jaguar than a three-toed sloth when losing fat.

By cycling periods of fasting, we allow the body to break down stored fat and convert it into fuel. This means there is more energy available to power the brain and body. With more resources available, we can keep our energy levels stable, so we no longer have to deal with the energetic mood swings of destructive dieting.

For years, they told us that a large carb-loaded breakfast was necessary to stay energised throughout the day. But this is not true. Doing the opposite and fasting instead will supply us with this long-lasting energy. Consistent energy levels provide a solid foundation upon which to build health and happiness. Not only will they increase your productivity, motivation and enjoyment of daily life, but losing fat also becomes rather effortless when you have energy. If you have more energy, you will move more and be more active, which will be of great help in managing the energy balance. When I say move more, I do not mean by exercise alone. There is another fundamental factor regarding losing fat and keeping it off, and it goes by the name of NEAT. **NEAT** stands for Non-Exercise Activity Thermogenesis, and it refers to the amount of energy we expend doing anything that *doesn't* involve sleeping, eating or structured exercise.

Walking the dog? NEAT.

Washing the car? NEAT.

Painting the bathroom? NEAT.

In fact, we could consider writing a positive review for this book as NEAT, given that research has shown typing to increase energy expenditure when compared to doing nothing. Although it may sound insignificant, NEAT matters, but we often neglect it. Let's imagine that you spend large periods of the day sitting down. If you were to swap the chair to stand up instead, you could increase the number of calories you burn throughout the day by up to 16%. A change like this alone could make all the difference in losing fat and keeping it off. While we're on the subject, let's break down what the total amount of energy expenditure may comprise on an average day by way of a pie chart.

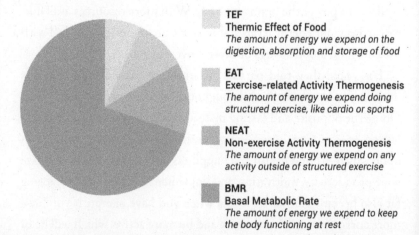

TEF
Thermic Effect of Food
The amount of energy we expend on the digestion, absorption and storage of food

EAT
Exercise-related Activity Thermogenesis
The amount of energy we expend doing structured exercise, like cardio or sports

NEAT
Non-exercise Activity Thermogenesis
The amount of energy we expend on any activity outside of structured exercise

BMR
Basal Metabolic Rate
The amount of energy we expend to keep the body functioning at rest

NEAT can make a huge difference. It's not all about focussing on our EAT and doing endless laps on the treadmill. Incorporating exercise is still something that I will always recommend, but it's not the *only* way. Have you ever gone hell for leather on a cardio machine, only to consult the screen afterwards and find out you only burned two hundred calories? I could consume two hundred calories within *seconds.*

The problem with relying on gruelling exercise to burn calories is that it may not be the most sustainable approach. When we push ourselves to do intense exercise, there is a certain *price* that we have to pay in terms of recovery. Periods of inactivity follow periods of exercise, and this will decrease the overall amount of NEAT. If you've given it all on the treadmill, then you're more likely to relax on the sofa and do less throughout the course of the day. We should not underestimate the difference this can make.

According to the research, staying active with NEAT is easier than adhering to an exercise program, and it may burn more calories. Dr. James Levine and his team at the Mayo Clinic found that, on average, energy expenditure from NEAT is larger than EAT over the course of the day. Further studies led them to conclude that focusing on increasing NEAT rather than EAT is a more sustainable strategy for losing fat and keeping it off. NEAT is variable, and the difference between sedentary and active individuals can be as much as one thousand calories a day. And if you can burn an extra thousand calories a day, then fat loss will be a breeze.

Prioritising those cardio sessions over everything else and spending the rest of the day moving at a snail's pace will not be the optimal approach. However, that's not to say that we should avoid exercise. Exercise has many benefits that transcend burning calories, and I encourage everyone to incorporate it into their lifestyle. I don't want to tell you that you need not exercise. I want to tell that you that increasing your daily activity can be just as effective as structured exercise in terms of fat loss, and perhaps easier to do. Let's consider Zug for a moment. Will Zug be exercising just for the sake of it? Probably not. He won't be sitting down at a desk for nine hours a day either. He will be on the move all throughout the day as he roams the savannah looking for food. So naturally he will maintain very high rates of NEAT. Increasing our daily activity in the form of NEAT is another way to emulate authentic patterns of human behaviour and make fat loss effortless. Outside of fat loss, attempting to be more active and increase NEAT will enhance the experience of daily life. And it may make you more charismatic too. Imagine two teachers. One of them is dynamic. Bouncing around the classroom and full of energy. The other is sedentary. Sitting down for the entire lesson on the verge of falling asleep. Which one will you learn more from? If you spend your working day on the move, not only will you *appear* more productive, you will *be* more productive too. People who are dynamic demand our respect. People who are passive and sedentary demand nothing. Increasing NEAT is emulating an authentic pattern of human behaviour, and it allows us to connect with the experience of being alive on a deeper level.

Exercise is beneficial, but relying on exercise alone to lose fat is a flawed approach. We should instead prioritise increasing our daily activity as much as possible. For example, modifying your desk so you can stand rather than sit. Walking to work instead of taking the bus. Or even just washing the dishes by hand. Perhaps in a million years, humans will have evolved to handle long periods of sitting down and the sedentary lifestyle. But at this stage in time, we are not designed for it. So avoid it wherever possible.

Introducing a little NEAT into your life makes constructing a healthy lifestyle a tidy job, but NEAT is a bit like *love*. The key to increasing NEAT for life is doing so without having to force it and letting it come naturally. Fasting is a great way to do this. Allow me to explain.

Burning stored fat for fuel helps to increase NEAT. But to dive further into the subject of fasting and NEAT, I must introduce an operative that you will not forget any time soon.

Orexin is a hormone that is primarily responsible for regulating wakefulness. While we are sleeping, orexin levels are low, but once we wake up and get going, they increase. When we stimulate orexin it leads to increased motivation, and a heightened sense of alertness. Scientists have associated higher levels of orexin with an increased rate of NEAT, as well as improved memory, motivation and mood. When we stimulate orexin, we feel more alert and motivated, so we move more and increase our NEAT. Stimulating orexin is an effective strategy in increasing NEAT and unlocking effortless fat loss. But where does fasting come into all of this?

Various studies show that fasting stimulates orexin. The brain perceives fasting as food scarcity, and it activates various survival mechanisms in response. Orexin is one of these mechanisms, as it makes us more alert, and therefore more likely to find food and survive the tough times.

The conventional wisdom that they have fed us over the years is that fasting will have a detrimental effect on energy levels. And we must eat at frequent intervals to maintain our energy levels. As we can see from the data, the conventional wisdom once again turns out to be nonsense. If we take this popular notion, that fasting makes a person feel lethargic, and frame it in an evolutionary context, it does not make sense.

Zug and his friends have gone a while without food and are feeling hungry. Alas, there are no supermarkets, no fast-food outlets and no fridge freezers around, so the only option is to find the food first hand. Not only that, but the conditions outside are rather harsh, and that sabre-toothed tiger over there looks rather peckish. Let's just imagine that Zug's energy levels and motivation were to deteriorate the longer he went without food. Would he be able to venture outside of the cave and find dinner, to end the food scarcity and survive? Probably not. And you and I would not be here today. How could humans have survived if we were to become *lazy* during times of food scarcity? We are the descendants of the hunter-gatherers that felt more energetic, alert, aware and motivated during periods of fasting and food scarcity. Because they were the ones who *survived*.

Everything comes down to survival. Rather than hamper our physical and mental capacities during periods of food scarcity and fasting, Mother Nature gives us a temporary physiological *upgrade*. Our life and the survival of the species depends on our ability to get out there and find food. The fact is that we *need* to be more alert and energetic during periods of fasting. For most of our time on earth, our life depended on it. The positive impact that fasting has on our alertness and energy levels is a survival mechanism that has allowed us to wander the planet for so long. Taking all of this into account, it seems absurd to think the overwhelming perception of fasting is that it will make a person tired and sluggish. But remember: Just because everyone says a thing is true, does not always make it so.

Despite what many people think, fasting increases energy levels. And because of this, it has a huge impact on NEAT, which scientists agree is an effective strategy for losing fat and keeping it off. Fasting encourages you to become more active throughout the day, helping to enhance the experience of life and manage the energy balance with ease.

Fasting gives us energy.

It's Mother Nature's pep talk.

SLEEPING
AND LIVING LONGER

*Sleep is the single most effective thing we can do to reset our brain
and body health each day -- Mother Nature's best effort yet at contra-
death.*

- MATTHEW WALKER

Fasting is not a panacea. It's a game-changer, but it's not magic. Sleep,
however, is a different matter. Good sleep is so beneficial that we may
as well classify it as a magical panacea. A good night's sleep can make
anything better, yet this modern society neglects it.

The younger me did not understand just how integral sleep is to
optimal health. Rarely would I sleep over six hours a night. And I
would often cut my sleep short to wake up at silly o'clock and get to
the gym before work. On average, I was sleeping between four and
five hours a night. I thought I was doing the right thing, but if only I
knew how destructive this really was. And how much it was holding
me back from reaching my goals. I was so dedicated and committed,
we should applaud this kind of behaviour, right?

Wrong. Neglecting sleep is a destructive habit.

If doing exercise before work means cutting one's sleep drastically
short, then it will always be a better idea to skip the exercise and stay
in bed. Don't worry about the societal norms and the flawed maxim
of 'just sleep when you're dead'. If you don't sleep, you *will* die. How's
that for a maxim? Quality sleep must always be a top priority, and
we ignore it at our peril. If we look at the data, the power of sleep
becomes clear. However, I warn you, if you are not familiar with the

science of sleep*, then the following information may shock you.

First, some context. In scientific terms, they consider an individual *sleep deprived* if they are sleeping less than six hours a night. That fact alone may shock many people who hate the alarm clock. I know it definitely shocked me when I first heard it. Regarding what the scientists would consider an optimal amount of sleep, it would seem that the cutoff point in the collective research is seven hours, below which adverse outcomes increase. Individual differences will always exist, but on average a minimum of seven hours of sleep a night should be the target. Don't let the people who say they can function with a few hours sleep fool you. Sleeping more is *always* worth it.

The effects of sleep deprivation are rather nuanced. That is to say that if you do not get enough sleep, your brain will work against you in subtle ways. Regarding fat loss, the research is clear. Sleep deprivation increases the risk of weight gain. Researchers from the University of Arizona found that better subjective sleep quality increased the likelihood of weight-loss success by 33%. Further research shows that sleeping habits are a strong predictor of fat loss in adults. One study showed that a higher incidence of sleep fragmentation, classified by the number of times someone wakes up throughout the night, led to a *lower rate* of fat loss. Poor sleep makes fat loss a struggle. But *why?*

It would be hard to imagine that sleeping more would cause fat loss if we did not change our diet. That wouldn't make sense. There must be some other variables at play. And this is where you see that the effects of poor sleep are rather nuanced, because through subtle changes, sleep deprivation leads us to eat more and move less.

Have you ever had an increased appetite after a poor night's sleep? Sleep deprivation raises ghrelin, so your appetite will be harder to control if you don't sleep enough. Various studies support the notion

---

*I highly recommend the excellent book *Why We Sleep* by Matthew Walker. Ironically, it's a real eye-opener.

of sleep influencing appetite, showing that sleep deprivation results in increased hunger and food intake. In fact, researchers from the University of Lübeck in Germany found that *one night* of sleep deprivation can increase hunger. One night is all it takes. Some people have been depriving themselves for years.

Poor sleep will make you hungrier, but it will also lower your rate of energy expenditure, shifting the body into a lower gear. You are now using less energy, so the body becomes lethargic, and the brain becomes foggy. Combine this with a heightened appetite, and you have a troublesome day ahead. Not only will you feel like eating more, but you will burn fewer calories and the brain will not have the energy to intervene with willpower.

Motivation and willpower are key factors in staying on track, and they will suffer without sleep. Sleep deprived people have lower levels of self-control, and most positive endeavours in life, including fat loss, require self-control. After a poor night's sleep, I struggle to make good decisions, and I always gravitate towards the unhealthy option. Junk food is most appealing after a restless night.

Sleep scientist Matthew Walker and his team at the University of California, Berkeley, explored this phenomenon in more detail. They wanted to see how sleep affects self-control around food, so they compared the behaviours of sleep deprived and well-rested participants when exposed to various food stimuli. Not only did the sleep-deprived have a stronger desire for high-calorie foods, but they also consumed more calories on average than the well-rested participants.

When you are sleep deprived, calorie dense and hyper-palatable foods become irresistible. And you will feel inclined to eat more. Therefore, it does not require a great deal of analysis to deduce that fat loss is an uphill struggle if you deprive yourself of sleep. Staying on track is easier if you sleep well.

Moreover, if you deprive yourself of sleep, you will be less active throughout the day. We touched on it earlier when discussing NEAT, but we can burn a significant amount of calories just by being slightly more active and less lethargic. Researchers from the University of Toronto found that sleep deprivation led participants to reduce their walking pace and report feeling much more tired. This lack of energy can then translate into a lack of motivation, and before you know it, you don't want to do *anything*. You will struggle to prepare a wholesome meal or get to the gym after work if you are not keeping your sleep in check. Various studies have shown that sleep-deprived individuals are much more inclined to go for the *easy* option rather than selecting a more challenging task. Sleep deprivation makes you stay inside the comfort zone. And this is never a good place to be. A good night's sleep could be the difference between choosing the easy option of ordering a calorie dense takeaway or buying ingredients and preparing a home-cooked meal. Cutting sleep short wreaks havoc on the best laid plans for fat loss. But it also comes with several other health risks.

Poor sleep makes you more sensitive to pain and stress. It undermines your cognitive ability, your memory and your physical performance. And it can also amplify the symptoms of anxiety and depression.

When we look at the long-term consequences, however, the picture gets even bleaker. Emerging research is clarifying the link between sleep deprivation and a range of neurodegenerative disorders, such as Alzheimer's disease. The data on sleep deprivation makes for grim reading, but the consensus is clear: if you deprive yourself of sleep, your risk of death increases. Now you can see the shortcomings of the popular mantra *just sleep when you're dead*. Because if you don't sleep, you will die. And it will not be peaceful. Sleep is vital for our overall health, but many people are unaware and deprive themselves under the illusion that sleep is not important.

When you deprive yourself of sleep, the body works against you. Mother Nature equipped you with the mechanisms to thrive during periods of food scarcity, but we cannot say the same for *sleep* scarcity. Humans have evolved with periods of food scarcity, but it is only with the work-obsessed modern society that we have introduced the concept of sleep scarcity. In 1910, the average person slept for 9 hours a night. Today, that average is down to 6.8 hours. Zug and the rest of our hunter-gatherer ancestors would not have been forcing themselves out of bed to make an early meeting. They would have been sleeping for as long as their body would allow and enjoying all the recovery time that they could.

Have you ever met someone who wears their lack of sleep like a medal, as if it's some kind of achievement or a symbol of their dedication?

'I only slept two hours last night. No one is more dedicated to this project than me.'

Sorry, Dave, you're still a moron. And you look like how a hangover feels.

When you look at the data, glorifying sleep deprivation is absurd, but it is prevalent in our work-obsessed culture. Good sleep is the cornerstone of any sustainable healthy lifestyle. Neglecting it comes with a hefty price tag and we do so at our peril. But there is some good news: sleeping more is easy, free and fun. Now we must ask, how can *fasting* affect our sleep?

A fasting lifestyle usually involves skipping the meal that you would eat first thing in the morning. Although some people may adjust their fasting window to accommodate for a morning meal, most people will fast for at least a few hours after waking up. Some may fast for even longer until the afternoon. But almost everyone who is fasting can afford a little more sleep in the morning now that they don't have to worry about breakfast. Similarly, a routine of daily fasting will prevent eating late at night. When you eat at night, you kick the digestive system back into action and the resulting hormonal activity can disrupt sleep and increase morning appetite. Eating a large meal before going to bed can also cause acid reflux and heartburn, which will not make for a peaceful slumber. If you are living the fasting lifestyle, then you will avoid the late night feast, and you will sleep better for it. Having a cut-off point in the evening to stop consuming calories allows the body to prepare itself for sleep. And on that note, it's time to introduce another hormone.

Melatonin regulates our sleep/wake cycle. When bedtime beckons, melatonin carries the signal to *power down* and prepares you for another night of sleep. Darkness releases melatonin, which is why exposure to screens late at night makes it harder to get to sleep. Optimal melatonin production is key for improving sleep quality and raising morning alertness, and many people who are struggling with sleep use it as a supplement. But it's still tricky to work out the optimal dosage. Luckily, melatonin has a working relationship with insulin. According to Dr. Elmar Peschke, who studied this relationship: 'an increase in melatonin levels leads to a down-regulation of insulin secretion and vice versa.' When you keep insulin low, you strengthen the melatonin signal, making it easier to get to sleep. This helps to explain the body of research that shows people with chronically elevated levels of insulin often have sleep issues. It also explains why eating late at night can disrupt sleep, as eating raises insulin.

A fasting lifestyle lowers insulin, which will strengthen the signal of melatonin. Therefore, incorporating fasting could be a small step towards improving your sleep. According to researchers from the Kliniken Essen Mitte hospital in Germany, a fasting lifestyle not only improves sleep but also enhances time spent awake. They found that participants who followed intermittent fasting for just one week improved their sleep quality and increased their levels of daytime performance.

The importance of sleep is undeniable. Realising this is the first step in making sure you get enough, but here are some additional guidelines that may also provide some value:

+ **Treat sleep as a top priority.**

No questions asked. This is about your health. And not just your physical health. Nobuaki Sakamoto and his team at the National Center for Global Health and Medicine in Tokyo, Japan wanted to see if there was a link between bedtimes and depression. They observed workers from the Furukawa Electric Corporation and found that those who went to bed later and slept less experienced more depressive symptoms. If someone messages or phones you late in the evening seeking a chinwag, then it must wait. Even if it's that special one. Swap the Netflix series for a couple more hours of sleep. It will pay dividends. Self love is a popular topic at the moment. If you want self love, then give yourself the gift of sleep. It is the highest form of self love.

+ **Avoid screens close to bedtime.**

Exposure to screens and lights at night makes it harder to get to sleep. When bedtime looms, remove all external stimuli and allow your mind and body to power down and prepare for a good night's sleep. If there is a screen present at bedtime, there is the danger of entering a rabbit hole and indulging in sleep procrastination. For example, let's say you plan to scroll for five minutes before bed. However, it goes for much longer than planned, and the next thing you know it's 3 am and you are on the weird side of YouTube. Remove the screen, remove the risk.

+ **Set aside half an hour to an hour before bedtime.**

Use it to take part in an activity that can make falling asleep easier. I recommend stretching and/or reading. Give yourself an hour before you go to sleep in which to disconnect from all distractions, stretch out a little, and then sink into something to read. Reading will help you sleep, but swapping the screen for a book has countless benefits that transcend sleep quality. Researchers from the University of Sussex found that reading reduced stress levels by 68%, which sounds like the perfect prelude to a good night's sleep. A study from the Yale University School of Public Health found that reading reduced mortality risk by 20%. Reading will improve your life. And even increase your chances of staying alive.

+ **Try to establish a regular bedtime.**

Researchers at the Sleep Science Center at the Taipei Medical University Hospital found that having an irregular bedtime schedule resulted in a worse night's sleep. Bedtime doesn't have to be an exact science, but aiming for a consistent bedtime on most days of the week is straightforward to do, and the benefits are huge.

Creating a healthy lifestyle requires a set of non-negotiables. These are your top priorities that are not up for debate. Giving yourself at least eight hours of *sleep opportunity* every night should be one of them. The term sleep opportunity refers to the time between getting into bed and getting out. In assuming that we are sleeping from the moment we get into bed to when we wake up, we often miscalculate how long it is that we are sleeping. Eight hours of sleep opportunity ensures that you will get at least seven hours of quality sleep. It's hard to do with the pressures and various obligations of modern life, but it *is* possible. Ensuring you get sufficient sleep will be easier with fasting too, as it removes distractions such as worrying about breakfast or struggling to eat something late at night.

If you sleep well, you will feel alert, happy and able to use your time much more efficiently than Dave, who still thinks sleeping four hours a night is admirable.

Cutting sleep short will *never* be worth it.

POSITIVITY, GRATITUDE, AND ACING THE TEST

People often ask me what I have for breakfast. The answer?
I have one less decision to make.

- SCOTT MURRAY

We do not associate destructive dieting with happiness. Fasting, however, makes you feel *good*. Even when losing fat.

Emerging clinical research shows fasting can improve mood levels in patients with depressive symptoms, but why is this?

PHYSIOLOGICAL

When you think of happiness, do serotonin and dopamine come to mind?

Serotonin and dopamine are important chemical messengers that regulate our mood and behaviour, and fasting may influence their activity.

Research links low serotonin with depression and anxiety, but it also regulates impulsive behaviour. One study from the University of Utah found that people with lower serotonin struggled to control their impulses around food. When you feel low, junk food becomes attractive, and the temptation to give in is overwhelming. Happiness keeps us on track.

When we consult the data, we see that fasting increases serotonin in rodents, but what about humans? To find out, researchers from Shahid Beheshti University of Medical Sciences in Iran measured levels of serotonin in participants at three different stages during the month of Ramadan. These stages were two days before Ramadan started, halfway through, and on the last day. By the halfway stage, levels of serotonin increased by 33%. By the end, the total increase was 43% when compared to the reading the researchers took before the start of the month. This appears to replicate the findings from animal research, but there are some limitations with this study. The main one being that those observing Ramadan are placing extra emphasis on *gratitude*. And gratitude, as we will see shortly, is key to cultivating happiness.

Although we associate dopamine with pleasure, emerging research shows that there is a lot more to the story. Many in the scientific community now refer to dopamine as the *motivation molecule*. When you lack dopamine, you lack motivation. Several mood disorders that involve diminished motivation, such as depression, usually involve a dopamine deficiency. Dopamine also plays a key role in learning, memory, cognition, and emotion. All key factors that we will need if we are going to act on our motivation. According to leading dopamine researcher Mercè Correa:

It was believed that dopamine regulated pleasure and reward and that we release it when we obtain something that satisfies us, but in fact the latest scientific evidence shows that this neurotransmitter acts before that, it actually encourages us to act. In other words, dopamine is released in order to achieve something good or to avoid something evil.

Achieving good and avoiding evil sound like perfect things for Zug to do during a period of food scarcity, which would explain why fasting stimulates dopamine production. The best time for us to feel motivated is when our life is on the line. When the brain stimulates dopamine, we feel motivated to explore our environment and learn more about it. Have you ever enjoyed a whole new level of perception while in the fasted state? When I'm fasting, I'm more aware of my surroundings. After incorporating fasting, some people say they notice things on their walk to work that they had never seen before. Consider this in the evolutionary framework. Would Zug require a little extra motivation and awareness when faced with a period of food scarcity? A boost in motivation would have been the catalyst for Zug to venture into the wild to find food. The elevated awareness and perception would have helped him to be more mindful of the environment and any potential threats or clues within it. Without the surge of dopamine during food scarcity, Zug may not have noticed the strange footprints in the mud or any other indications that would lead to food or warn of predators. Without the boost in motivation, Zug may have instead opted to stay in the comfort of the warm cave, and we would not be here today.

Outside of serotonin and dopamine, there may be another physiological reason for the positive vibes that come with fasting. As we discussed earlier in the book, you produce ketone bodies as a fuel source when you break down stored fat during periods of fasting. Various studies have associated these ketone bodies with improvements in mood and a sense of wellbeing, but just ask anyone in ketosis* how they are feeling. Without a doubt, they will have something positive to say.

Let's take Sandy, for example.

After not seeing Sandy for almost the whole season, I bumped into him at a football match towards the end of the campaign. He looked well, but he told me that not so long ago, the doctor diagnosed him as pre-diabetic†. As a result, his forward-thinking doctor prescribed him a regimen of fasting and a ketogenic way of eating to turn things around. In all the years I've known Sandy, he has always been going on about how something would impede him painting the fence in his

---

*a metabolic state characterized by raised levels of ketone bodies in the body.

†we will be exploring pre-diabetes in great detail in chapter five.

back garden. As is turns out, it was being in ketosis that motivated Sandy to get off his backside and get painting. Not only that, but he was *singing* while he did it too.

GRATITUDE

If you have ever struggled to focus on the positive rather than the negative, then I would not worry. You are not alone. We *all* do it. And that's because it's what Mother Nature designed us to do as humans. It's called the Negativity Bias. There could be countless positives in life, but as soon as one little negative turns up, it demands up all of our attention.

It's a survival mechanism. She built us to do this.

How long would an extreme optimist survive in the wild?

Being sceptical and thinking of the negatives was helpful back when we were wearing rags. More than anything, it kept us alive. The survival of Zug and our ancestors depended on their ability to approach situations with a mindset that considered the worst-case scenario. This allowed them to sidestep any potential danger. Back when we roamed the African Savannah, we had to prioritise the negative over the positive to identify potential threats, avoid them, and therefore survive. Throughout our evolution, this was a useful trait, and it has served a purpose as we are still here today. When faced with a broad spectrum of predators and harmful situations, we require a pessimistic eye to avoid danger. However, today everything is different. And these same survival systems that once kept us alive are now not so beneficial. Now that our survival is all but secured, we focus on negatives that have no right to detract from the vast array of positives we enjoy daily. I often hear people complaining about trivial matters, such as the weather or the fact that Dave ate the last biscuit in the break room. But I rarely hear them express gratitude for the good things in life. Of which there are many.

All a bit silly, isn't it?

Gratitude is how you will overcome the negativity bias.

If you are expressing gratitude for the good in life, it's hard to focus on the bad. But it's tough to do. Expressing gratitude requires effort. As the old saying goes: 'absence makes the heart grow fonder'. The best way to appreciate something is to go without it. Maybe you have to move away to realise how much you love your family. Or go camping in the rain to realise how amazing it is to have a warm bed and clean sheets. To appreciate eating, we have to spend some time *fasting*. Fasting is a great way to practice gratitude and beat the negativity bias. By cycling periods of fasting and feeding, it's difficult *not* to feel grateful when it's time to break the fast. This is in stark contrast to when I would eat all day and never reflect on what a privilege it is to eat whenever I like. Fasting blesses us with some much-needed perspective. And as we mentioned earlier, it heightens our perception too, so when you're fasting, take a walk outside. You may just discover a newfound gratitude for nature.

Fasting makes you feel grateful, helping to shift focus away from the negative and onto the positive. It could also make you more savvy in your decision-making.

DECISION FATIGUE

Decision fatigue is a psychological concept referring to the decline in cognitive abilities after having to make too many decisions. As more and more decisions confront us through the day, our mental capabilities dwindle, and it becomes harder to make the right choice.

Decision fatigue plays a role in many areas of life, including fat loss. Building a healthy lifestyle requires good decisions, because good choices lead to further good choices. However, poor judgement leads to more poor judgement, which is why many people can go off track after one bad decision. Maybe you know someone who made one poor choice that led to them losing control. Minimizing decision fatigue helps us to stay on track.

In 2016, Danish psychologist Hans Henrik Sievertsen and his team wanted to see if the time of the day impacted student performance on a test.

On average, students that took the test first thing in the morning performed better than the students that took the test later on in the day. In the morning, the students were fresh and able to make the right choices. But as the day wore on, and they accumulated decision fatigue, their test performance suffered. Our ability to make good decisions is a *finite* resource. The more decisions we have to make, the worse our judgement gets. Decision fatigue plays a significant role in the outcome of the choices we make. Let's imagine you have arrived at home following a long day full of decisions. At this stage, your brain is too fatigued to think about what you should cook. So you shove a pizza in the oven, open a beer, and round it all off with some ice cream. Decision fatigue makes fat loss a struggle, and it subtracts from our quality of life.

The beauty of fasting lies in its *simplicity*. It's easy to fall into the trap of complicating our lives to get healthier and happier, but simplicity is beautiful. There are many voices in this world that encourage us to add more things because it benefits them and their profit margin. In reality, we need very little. And most of it we already have. Fasting is subtraction, not addition, and this opens a whole new avenue of freedom. For example, rather than stress about sourcing a healthy breakfast or worry about where you can eat lunch on a business trip, you can just fast. If you have a busy day ahead, you can lighten the mental load with fasting. If you can minimise decision fatigue with fasting, it also means that when the time arrives to eat, you are fresher and ready to make good choices regarding your nutrition.

Fasting reduces the amount of decisions we have to make, which allows us to make them with a higher level of clarity.

And better decisions make for a better life.

SUSTAINABILITY

Sometimes greatness is the result of a transcendent, peak performance.
But often, greatness is simply the result of a good performance
repeated and sustained much longer than usual.

- JAMES CLEAR

Have you ever struggled to find something to eat in the airport that didn't require taking out a mortgage to have any hope of purchasing it?

I have.

Have you ever gone out to dinner and gazed at the menu in fear, worrying about what you would eat?

I have.

Have you ever spent too much time worrying about whether something is healthy?

I have.

In attempting to get healthy, have you ever developed an unhealthy relationship with food, and even yourself?

I know I have.

Fast forward to the present day, and fasting has eliminated a lot of worry from my life. I don't have to worry about finding something to eat at the airport anymore, because I can just fast. I don't have to worry about my appetite anymore, because fasting allows me to eat big satisfying meals, and it controls my hunger when I'm not eating. I don't have to worry about what I will eat if I go out to a restaurant anymore, because fasting for most of the day gives me calorie freedom.

When I needed saving, fasting answered the call. And it has improved my life immeasurably. But that's just my experience. What about everyone else?

Making healthy changes is a great idea. But unless you can maintain them as part of a lifestyle, they will be worthless. Sustainability is the key word here. So we must ask: is intermittent fasting sustainable? And it's impossible to give a black and white answer. In reality, it is highly nuanced, as it depends on the individual and their circumstances. However, I believe intermittent fasting *is* sustainable. And let me tell you why. It gets easier with time until it becomes second nature. It gives you calorie freedom, which will enhance your social life and your enjoyment of food. It simplifies your everyday life and eliminates a lot of worries. And it makes you feel *good*, as opposed to destructive dieting. Which makes you feel *miserable*.

When I was a child, my favourite thing by far was Lego. Let's imagine you have some building blocks, and you have to build a strong structure. When you build with simple blocks, you can build strong structures. However, when you build with complicated pieces, the result is fragile. Starting with drastic restrictions and deprivation makes for a fragile structure and going slightly off track has the power to destroy it. When it crumbles, you are back at square one. Intermittent fasting is a primitive building block. It is super simple, and it lends itself to many other simple blocks. Once you start fasting, you become more active. You sleep better. You drink more water and avoid liquid calories. You become more in touch with your authentic appetite. You can enjoy your social life. You strengthen your interpersonal relationships. You feel love. You feel alive. And these are all fundamental parts of a healthy lifestyle.

Start with fasting, and before you know it, you have a stable structure in place.

And this will lead to long-term fulfilment and happiness.

Part Three

YOUR FASTING LIFESTYLE

Fasting is a game changer, but where do you start?
Luckily, it's simple.

No drastic dietary changes,
fat-burning pills,
or monthly subscriptions are required.

THE RULES, RISKS, AND GETTING STARTED

That which does not kill us makes us stronger.

- FRIEDRICH NIETZSCHE

Fasting is safe. If it was not, Zug would not have survived. However, modern life is not so simple.

You should *not* be fasting if:

+ You are pregnant.
+ You are breastfeeding
+ You are diabetic
+ You are taking medication and have not consulted your doctor.
+ You are under 18 years of age
+ You are underweight and/or struggle to gain weight
+ You have gone to extreme lengths to lose weight in the past
+ You have a history of disordered eating
+ You have a chronic disease

If there are any doubts, always consult your doctor.

Fasting is a healthy process, but it can create unhealthy situations. If problems arise with fasting, it is usually the fault of these various situations. To further explain this point, let's refer to Person X.

Despite being at a healthy weight, Person X has always struggled with their image and never enjoyed a healthy relationship with food. They have subscribed to every destructive dieting tactic in the book and will regularly go to extreme lengths to lose weight. Upon discovering the concept of fasting, Person X takes it to the limit. On some days, they will fast for almost the entire day yet still deprive themselves during the feeding window. On other days, they will just try to fast for as long as they can. Person X is using fasting to mask an underlying eating disorder, and this is something we must always be aware of.

Fasting makes it easier to eat less. It regulates our appetite and controls the energy balance, which is beneficial for the vast majority of people. However, it can be problematic for those who are prone to going to extreme lengths to lose weight or have a history of disordered eating. Fasting can exacerbate a poor relationship with food because it places additional restrictions on eating. Eating disorder experts agree that eating behaviours involving excessive restriction or rigid rules can be a precursor to diagnosable eating disorders. For the vast majority of people looking to make healthy changes, some form of restriction is essential. But for those who have struggled with an unhealthy relationship with food or disordered eating in the past, applying additional restrictions to their eating behaviours can develop into destructive habits. This scenario is rare, but we must take it into consideration. With that said, there are cases where people have overcome eating disorders with fasting. This is also rare, but it does occur. One thing that we can say for sure is that we must always exercise flexibility. Fasting is not synonymous with deprivation. It is a tool that we can use to enhance our enjoyment of food and of everyday life. If it starts to drift from this purpose, then take a moment to reassess.

STRESS

It is important to remember that fasting is a *stressor*. Now, I know what you're thinking:

'Isn't stress bad?'

And the answer is: it depends.

Excessive or chronic stress can lead to serious health complications, but manageable doses are beneficial. We need a certain amount of stress for growth, and this is a concept known as hormesis.

> *Hormesis is one of those words that most people don't know,*
> *representing a concept that they do.*
> *Once you name it, you see the pattern everywhere, in biology and*
> *psychology, systems and civilizations.*
>
> - NAVAL RAVIKANT

Derived from the Greek word *hormo*, which means to excite or stimulate, hormesis is a biological phenomenon whereby exposure to manageable doses of stress results in beneficial adaptations. As Naval said, once you know the name, you will see hormesis everywhere. It is hormetic stress that underpins all kinds of growth, development and learning. A great example of hormesis is building muscle. Resistance training applies stress to the muscle tissue that breaks it down. When you are training at the gym, you are not growing bigger; you are doing the exact opposite and breaking the muscles down. But this stress is a necessary stimulant for growth. Applying the stress of weight training breaks down muscle tissue, but it challenges it to grow back bigger and stronger. Without the hormetic stress of resistance training, the muscles would never have a reason to grow. Excessive weight training above and beyond what we require for growth will do more harm than good, and this is where we see the sweet spot. Hormetic stress is all about balance. The dose is important. Adversity brings out the best of us, and stress helps us to grow, but too much of it can burn a person out. The key to optimal health is balancing stressors.

Fasting operates with a similar principle. It is a stressor to the system, but we can harness the stress and use it to our benefit. The body can rise to the challenge and thrive. What we must be mindful of when implementing fasting is the *total* amount of stressors in our life. Fasting is not problematic, but the manner in which it interacts with other factors in our life *can* be. If a person is training hard but neglecting their recovery, getting insufficient sleep, and experiencing stress at work, then adding in the stressor of fasting is not a good idea.

Fasting is a stressor. Whether we can utilise it to our benefit or it has a negative impact depends on the other factors at play in our lifestyle.

GROUND RULES

- We do not consume any calories during the fasting period.
- Acceptable liquids are water, black coffee and green tea.
- Drink plenty of water.
- Always remember to be flexible. Fasting is a tool, not a prison.

Easy.

GETTING STARTED

When we first incorporate fasting into our life, there are two distinct paths we can take. Either we can jump straight into the deep end, or we can ease into it.

I jumped straight into it. Working long hours made it easy.

Back then, I arrived at work early and couldn't leave until around midnight, but I had a long break during the day (hospitality. Say no more). Eating before work made me feel sluggish, and eating late at night after I got home disrupted my sleep. Because of this predicament, I ate only within the break that sandwiched itself between lunch and dinner. This meant I wouldn't have to squeeze in a big meal between the gym and going to work in the morning. And I could just go straight to sleep upon arriving home at night. As a result, I was fasting for an average of 20 to 22 hours a day from the get-go. On my days off, I would naturally extend my feeding window to accommodate for social events. I wasn't adhering to a concrete fasting schedule every single day; rather I was being flexible and using fasting as a tool to make my life easier. This approach may sound extreme to some, but I loved it from the first minute. I was desperate for a change, which helped, but it also simplified my life and saved me a lot of time. Not to mention how sharp I felt. However, the circumstances I found myself in and my experience are unique, so we must consider alternative methods.

A more gentle approach would be to ease into the groove of fasting. It's important to remind ourselves of what our aim is. We don't want a quick fix. We want a *lifestyle*. Therefore, it makes sense to take our time to get accustomed to fasting. Although I think it is unlikely, rushing into fasting may prove too difficult for some, which could then put them off fasting entirely. Remember, it's a lifestyle change. Fasting will be around for a very long time, so there is no rush to implement it.

My first recommendation is to establish a time in the evening to stop consuming calories altogether. This is a great exercise in discipline, and it serves to extend the natural overnight fasting period of our sleep. Once this becomes natural, consider pushing the first meal of the day back further. This step will be straightforward for those who are not so keen on breakfast or who lack time in the mornings. Start with an hour delay and extend it over the next few days or weeks until the fasting period reaches the desired length. Fasting should soon become an *effortless* affair. Many people find that implementing a set time in the evening to stop eating alone is effective in terms of fat loss. This is because we mainly consume foods easy to overindulge in, like sweets and crisps, during the later hours when the sofa and television beckon. Sustainability is the key word here, so take everything step by step. People who try to accomplish multiple goals are less committed and less likely to succeed than those who focus on just a single goal. Set a small goal and focus on seeing it through to completion. Once accomplished, set a new one, and repeat the process. Greatness awaits.

Almost everything in life gets easier with time and practice. Fasting is no exception.

The more you do it, the more effortless it becomes, and before you know it, fasting will be like second nature. The first few weeks can be tough for some. There can be headaches and feelings of fatigue, but these are withdrawal symptoms and should dissipate within a week.

Above all, remain patient and stay strong.

The first few weeks will always be hard, but it's worth it.

FEMALES WHO FAST

I think women are foolish to pretend they are equal to men, they are far superior and always have been.

- WILLIAM GOLDING

Females are amazing. But women of the world, I have some bad news. You will have more fat than men. It will be harder to lose. And it will take more time. Your physiology will push back harder. But there is always a solution.

Evolution demands that females carry more fat than men. Between menstruation and menopause, Mother Nature designed the female to produce babies, so there has to be more energy in reserve. This is something that is often overlooked. And it is also somewhat ironic if we consider that, according to the research, women will go to greater lengths to lose weight than men. Therefore, women will often subscribe to destructive and drastic dieting. But this can come with several downsides. When females diet down to low levels of body fat, they often lose their menstrual cycle and experience a broad range of hormonal problems. The astronomical beauty standards of this hyper-connected world set unrealistic expectations. And the price of chasing them is high. However, it is important to remember many people we see on social media are not playing by the rules.

We are living in an age where there are more women taking anabolic steroids than ever before. This allows them to build more muscle, lose more fat, and manipulate their menstrual cycle. They then post the fruits of their labour to their online highlight reel. What they do with their life is their business. But they are setting unrealistic expectations of what is naturally possible for many people, whether they know it or not. Looking perfect is profitable. If you can make people feel inadequate, you can sell them supplements, destructive dieting plans, and other worthless piffle. But this is not reality. So be vigilant with how you scroll.

Moving on, whether females should incorporate fasting generates much debate. Various sources claim they should not as it can disrupt their hormones and lead to fertility problems, but this is not the case.

I struggle to see how intermittent fasting, which is essentially giving yourself an extended break between meals, could be so problematic. It would seem like a rather healthy process. Regardless, there is still a concern. And if concern remains, then we must address it, so let's get right into it. I am not a woman myself, so rather than refer to my experience with fasting, I will have to rely on the data available.

In 2016, Dr. Pradeep M. K. Nair, a researcher for the Indian government, set out to examine what kind of role therapeutic fasting can play in female health. After reviewing the data, he found nothing to suggest that fasting could have a *negative* impact. He did, however, find research suggesting that fasting could reduce the symptoms of Polycystic Ovary Syndrome (PCOS). PCOS is a condition with symptoms ranging from a mild menstrual disorder to a severe disturbance of reproductive functions. If we were to rely on the data alone, then we might assume that fasting is safe for females, but this would be a flawed approach.

The first reason for this would be because we are working with a small data set. Second, life is not always so black and white. There is always a multitude of variable factors at play in each individual case that can affect the outcomes. Regardless of what conclusions we can glean from the data, there must be some women out there who have experienced problems with fasting. If not, we would not be having this discussion.

I have met females that found fasting problematic. But I have also encountered females who love it. I even met one lady who restored her menstrual cycle after incorporating intermittent fasting. Anecdotal evidence does not make the rule, but it seems to go both ways. Let's consider all the possibilities and talk about what we know. We know that drastic calorie restriction, nutritional deficiencies, sudden weight loss, excessive exercise and stress are all factors that disrupt the female hormonal balance. They can impact the menstrual cycle and trigger problems such as hair loss. The question is: does fasting have the potential to promote any of these factors?

FOOD FOR THOUGHT

Incorporating fasting can affect overall nutrient intake, which is a factor in the female hormonal balance.

Many people associate cutting out carbohydrates with optimal health and weight loss. Some will see fantastic results from carbohydrate reduction or from following a ketogenic diet. Low-carb and ketogenic ways of eating come with a plethora of health benefits, and they have helped many people to lose weight who had struggled before. But there is no black and white in nutrition. Studies on the subject of low-carbohydrate diets and females paint a mixed picture. Some women will thrive on a low-carb diet, while others may encounter problems. What works for *everyone*, however, is managing the energy balance. Assuming that we can manage the energy balance, we can facilitate fat loss while still consuming carbohydrates. Cutting carbs can be beneficial, but it is not compulsory.

Problems arise when people change everything all at once. They implement fasting, cut out all carbs and join the gym on the same day. It's a lot of stress for the system to handle, and it can have consequences. Take things slow and steady.

Protein is the most satisfying macronutrient, so foods rich in protein are filling. You rarely hear of people binging on steaks. Some people struggle to consume enough protein within a feeding window. And this can be problematic as protein wears several hats. Not only is it responsible for maintaining muscle mass, but also in keeping our skin, nails and hair beautiful. Dietary protein is the building block of healthy hair. Protein deficiency can cause hair loss and hair thinning in females, so this is something that we must be mindful of when incorporating fasting and planning our nutrition. If protein intake is being sacrificed to adhere to a fasting schedule, then it is time to reassess the situation. Nutrition first, fasting later.

Protein is *satiating*. When we eat it, we feel *full*. For example, eating 500 calories of lean chicken breast will be much more filling than 500 calories of chocolate. This explains why it's hard to consume enough protein during a feeding window, but it also explains why protein consumption can have a positive impact on *leptin* activity. Leptin is responsible for the satisfaction signal, but it also plays a role in regulating the menstrual cycle, with research showing that very low leptin can cause irregular menstruation. Fat cells produce leptin and levels fall during periods of fasting. For females with moderate to high levels of body fat, the fasting-induced decrease of leptin is nothing to worry about. However, for the females with *low* levels of body fat, decreasing leptin during long periods of fasting may have some adverse effects regarding the menstrual cycle. For the lean ladies out there, it will be wise to avoid frequent long fasting periods. It will always depend on the individual, but it is something to consider. Remember, Mother Nature has tasked the female with bearing children, and does not want the female to lose too much body fat. Intuitively, it makes sense that low protein intake may interfere with the menstrual cycle. Dietary protein provides the building blocks to construct new connective tissue. If there is not enough protein, the female body would have to delay the construction project of the most important connective tissue of all: a child.

Remember, the body is resourceful and always adapting to the energy availability of an ever-changing environment.

Intermittent fasting itself is not problematic, but it can amplify some negative situations. Like I said, I have encountered some women who have experienced problems with fasting. But whenever we would sit down together and break down the whole situation piece by piece, it became apparent that there was something else going on. This would involve drastic calorie reduction, a very low protein intake, or a sudden drop in weight, which are all factors that can impact the female hormonal balance. To help shed light on this, let's refer to Brenda's story.

Brenda has recently started intermittent fasting and found that she has little to no appetite. This results in her eating much less than before and struggling to consume an adequate amount of protein. On top of this, she has also added more HIIT training to her routine and is not a fan of taking a rest day from the gym. As time passes, she feels a little strange and experiences some problems. Immediately, she concludes that it *must* be because of the fasting, and she does not hesitate to relegate intermittent fasting to the division of fad diets.

But hold on a second. What about everything else?

What about the drastic calorie reduction, the sudden drop in weight, the low protein intake, the excessive exercise or the increased amount of stressors to the system? We *know* that these are factors that can cause complications, but Brenda did not even consider them.

The fasting didn't do it; it merely contributed to creating an environment in which the harmful elements could flourish. Take a balanced approach with fasting, nutrition and exercise. And always consider all the factors.

THE MENSTRUAL CYCLE

Regarding female fitness and nutrition, the menstrual cycle is often overlooked, but it plays a very important role.

We can divide the menstrual cycle into three phases. The follicular phase makes up the first two weeks, ovulation is the middle point, and the luteal phase covers the last two weeks.

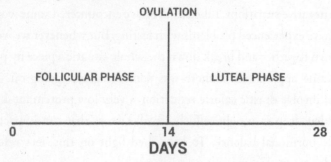

Female behaviour can vary dramatically during the cycle. You may have even found yourself on the receiving end of one of these variations. This is because of two hormones: estrogen and progesterone.

The estrogen hormones are the good guys during the menstrual cycle, as they reduce appetite and increase energy levels.

Estrogen is good news. But progesterone is a bit of a downer. It sends sugar cravings wild, saps energy and makes women feel miserable during menstruation. These two hormones affect behaviour, so let's look at how *they* behave during the menstrual cycle.

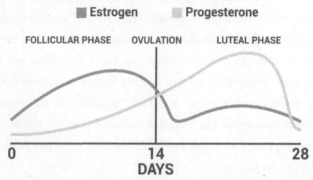

As you can see, there is a clear pattern. During the first two weeks, estrogen is high and progesterone is low. At ovulation, there is a crossover, with estrogen decreasing and progesterone going in the opposite direction. In the second stage of the cycle, progesterone is high and estrogen is low, which explains why the last two weeks are often the hardest.

In my experience of working with female clients, I have noticed two important factors regarding the menstrual cycle. The first is that females perform better in the gym during the first two weeks of their cycle. This improvement in performance and strength peaks at ovulation, at the middle of the cycle, at which point it declines. The second common theme is that things get a little pear-shaped in the last two weeks of the cycle. Females report having more cravings and less energy. They find it hard to resist temptation and struggle to find the motivation to go to the gym. We can assume this is because of the sharp increase in progesterone that we see in the luteal phase.

Hormonal changes throughout the menstrual cycle cause various fluctuations. Behaviour, mood, and appetite can all change with little to no notice. Another factor that is especially susceptible to fluctuation is *body weight*. This can get many women down. When they see the scale going in the wrong direction, they may feel like resorting to destructive dieting to resolve the situation. But this is not the way. It is just part of the cycle. For example, during the luteal phase, the body will hold on to more water weight, which can lead to some undesirable numbers on the scale. However, this does not mean that progress has stopped or that destructive dieting is necessary; it is just a natural part of the journey.

So what about fasting? The key to long-term success with intermittent fasting lies in *flexibility*. In the first two weeks of the cycle, staying on track is simple. During the follicular phase, energy is high and appetite is easy to control. The first two weeks are fine, but some find it hard to stay on track during the last two weeks of the cycle. In the luteal phase, hunger, cravings, and laziness can disrupt the best-laid plans for a healthy lifestyle. Having a fasting system in place can be key for staying on track during these final two weeks. Research shows that insulin sensitivity decreases during the luteal phase, explaining the surge in sugar cravings. Intermittent fasting is Mother Nature's very own insulin sensitiser, which helps to bring cravings under control. But it is also helpful in controlling appetite and elevating energy levels. Therefore, having a fasting system in place can help to avoid any potential banana skins during the luteal phase. However, it is also possible that during these last two weeks the body does not respond well to fasting. It is perhaps more sensitive to stress at this stage. And because fasting is a stressor, it may not be a comfortable combination. Therefore, you will need to listen to your body and learn how it responds at every stage.

Earlier, we mentioned how weight can fluctuate during the menstrual cycle, which leads to a great deal of frustration. To avoid the negativity, and to gain clarity over what is happening, I recommended tracking progress (with weight, progress photos, and body measurements) every week. But only compare changes once a month. For example, comparing your weight on week one of the cycle to week two of the same cycle will not be the optimal approach, given the fluctuations. A superior method of gauging progress is to compare week one to week one of the following cycle. Week two with the following week two, and so on and so forth. We can also take a similar approach with fasting. Consider how you feel with fasting at each stage of the cycle. Perhaps during the first two weeks, fasting is a breeze. But it is a struggle in the last two weeks. Compare your week one to the following week one, and you will gain a lot more clarity on how to plan your fasting schedule around the cycle.

With all things considered, there will always be individual differences. Some women struggle during certain points of the cycle. Others may not even notice it. Take things step by step, study how your body responds at various stages, and adapt accordingly.

SUMMARY

- Don't implement several changes at the same time. If you try to do everything all at once, it becomes very difficult to isolate what change is having what effect. Changing everything overnight will lead to confusion, stress, and frustration. Take it one step at a time.

- Don't obsess over the numbers. If you break your fast a little earlier than usual, it won't make a difference.

- Prioritise protein in your nutrition. If you are struggling to eat enough, then extend the feeding window. The exact quantities will depend on the individual, but making it a priority is always a good idea.

- More time spent fasting is not always better. And this is especially true for females with low levels of body fat. Long-term success lies in establishing the balance between fasting and feeding. Not in fasting for as long as possible.

- Always be flexible. Don't feel like you *have* to fast for the same time every single day. You don't.

- Your health and quality of life are much more important than adhering to a precise fasting protocol. If fasting subtracts from your quality of life, then take a moment to rethink your approach.

Females should start slow. The best course of action is to ease into it and assess how you feel at every step of the way. If you encounter any problems, take a step back and consider all the other lifestyle factors, such as diet and sleep, that may affect the overall picture. Females are more sensitive to weight loss and stress, so take gradual steps. Intermittent fasting gets a lot of negative press. Especially for the female. But we need not fear it. Fasting *itself* is not problematic. Rather, it is the environment it *can* create and the behavioural patterns that it *can* exacerbate that *may* cause problems. As long as you take it step by step and keep it balanced, you will be fine.

THE FASTING SCHEDULE AND RIDING THE HUNGER WAVE

The idea that "change is hard" is one of the biggest myths
about human behavior.
The truth is, you change effortlessly and all the time.
The primary job of the brain is to adjust your behavior
based on the environment. Design a better environment.
Change will happen naturally.

- JAMES CLEAR

How long should I fast for? It depends on your lifestyle.
Is there something special about a sixteen hour fast? Not really.
These are accurate answers, but they are also vague. Let's roll our sleeves up and get right into it.

The most popular method of incorporating fasting is to follow an intermittent pattern of a sixteen hour fasting window alongside a eight-hour feeding window. Most people will place this eight hour feeding window between noon and eight in the evening. Rather than sixteen being a magic number to fast or eating from midday to eight p.m. being optimal, the popularity of this approach comes from the convenience. Essentially, it is skipping breakfast and tightening things up in the evening, which is easy to do for most people. On a physiological level, we enter the fasted state twelve hours from our last meal. Therefore, sixteen hours will allow for the body to metabolise some stored energy and give the digestive system a break. There is nothing inherently special about sixteen hours of fasting, it just allows for a balance between fasting and feeding that suits most people. Do not feel you have to follow the same approach. And don't feel you have to adhere to a rigid schedule every single day.

Let's mix it up a little.

You can fast for sixteen hours of the day, but you can also fast for twelve or even twenty-three. Eating between noon and eight p.m. might suit your lifestyle, but maybe a feeding window of nine a.m. to five p.m. is more compatible, or perhaps even six till nine. Some days you can fast for longer, and on other days you can extend the feeding window. Some days you might fast, whereas other days you might not. The key to creating a healthy lifestyle is to exercise flexibility and find the balance. Doing the same thing every single day may work for some people, but for most, it is not a sustainable approach. Fasting is a tool that can enhance your enjoyment of food and of life, so let's make sure you are using it correctly.

Flexibility is crucial, and I believe one of the most flexible approaches to fasting is to tie the schedule to *events* rather than specific times. A few years ago, I set myself a feeding window of four p.m. to eight p.m., and I often watched the clock until it struck four. This habit subtracted from my quality of life, so I decided instead to schedule my fast according to events rather than the clock. For example, I decided that I would break my fast once I had completed my work for the day and had arrived home from the gym. Some days this would work out to be 4 p.m. on the dot, but other days it was a little later or even a little earlier. My fasting followed a similar pattern as before, but it never caught me clock-watching, and I was a lot more productive. Likewise, I would close my feeding window once food had satisfied me. Some days this would be after my main meal, but on some occasions, it required a little more. There were other days when there was a delay in preparing my food, so naturally, I would finish a little later on. I will not deprive myself of dinner just because I have passed a certain point of clock time. That sounds absurd, and it is, but many people do it. The benefit of this approach was that I never had to worry about the time. As a result, I could develop a natural rhythm of fasting and feeding perfectly in sync with my lifestyle. This is a philosophy that I believe can be applied to many other areas of life too. Judging the trajectory of our life according to clock time is not the way to long-term fulfilment. Using events and experiences as a metric is much more useful.

Regarding the timing of the fasting schedule, don't worry about the small differences. In the grand scheme of things, it does not matter.

What is the optimal time to fast? It depends on several factors.

First, fat burning does not always equate to fat *loss*. Burning fat for fuel through fasting can be a very useful tool for many reasons, but if we overeat in the feeding window, it will not result in fat loss. If I eat my bodyweight in Jaffa Cakes and exceed my energetic needs during the feeding window, fasting will be irrelevant, because fat loss will not be on the agenda. Remember, plenty of people have lost fat and will continue to do so *without* the use of fasting. We still need to nail the fundamentals. The optimal time to fast, therefore, is whatever time frame suits *you* and allows *you* to sustain a fasting schedule as part of a healthy and enjoyable lifestyle.

Keep it simple and don't get hung up on the minutiae[*].

---

[*]minutiae means the small, precise, or trivial details of something. It's a great word.

Embrace fasting for the tool it is and use it accordingly. Andy, a friend of mine, is not massively keen on daily fasting. However, if Andy has a big dinner coming up, he will fast before, as this gives him calorie freedom and allows him to enjoy his night. Likewise, if Andy has a busy day on the cards, he does not panic. He knows that he can pull the fasting tool out of his locker and use it to be more productive. When it's time to travel, Andy knows that, rather than having to find good food in the airport and on the plane, he can just fast, and this makes him happy. If Andy is feeling particularly inflamed* or struggling with a digestive issue, he will utilise fasting to help soothe the symptoms. Andy does not fast every day, but he recognises that fasting is a useful tool that he can use in a plethora of potentially tricky situations. However, not everyone is like Andy, and many people want to incorporate fasting as part of a lifestyle. To further explain how to do so, I will refer to a friend of ours we met at the beginning of the book. Remember Mo?

Mo works at a busy Irish pub in the touristic quarter of Barcelona. On a typical day, Mo wakes up at noon, starts work at seven p.m., has a break at ten and finishes at around one thirty in the morning. Recently, Mo has become distressed and finds it difficult to adhere to a feeding window of noon til eight p.m. with his lifestyle. It means that he has to eat as soon as he wakes up and go to the gym on a full stomach. And there is nothing to look forward to eating during his break at work. I asked Mo why he feels like he has to adhere to this schedule. His response: *well, that's what everyone else is doing.*

But Mo is not everyone else. He is Mo, and he has his own preferences and lifestyle factors that he must take into consideration when planning the fasting schedule.

Remember, the *total* time that we spend fasting is the important factor. If Terry stops eating at six p.m. on one day and starts again

---

*more on fasting and inflammation in part six.

at ten a.m. the next, he has fasted for sixteen hours. Likewise, if Mo stops eating at eleven p.m. and starts again at three p.m. the following day, he is still fasting for sixteen hours, just between different times to Terry. To put it poetically, it doesn't matter *when* you do it, as long as you *do* it. The specific times in which you fast depend on your preference, so find a schedule compatible with your lifestyle and crack on. I suggested to Mo that he adjust his feeding window so he could begin eating at three p.m. and aim to finish by eleven. That way, he doesn't have to eat as soon as he wakes up, which he prefers. Instead, Mo can exercise his beloved *fasted power* in the gym and work up an appetite for a big break-fast before he has to get ready for work. Not having to worry about eating liberates some time, so Mo can complete any outstanding errands before he goes to work. This means Mo's average day always begins productively, so when he sits down for his break-fast meal, he does not have to rush. It also affords Mo the time to prepare a big wholesome meal at home. The leftovers of which he then can take to work later and avoid the distractions of fast food indulgence during his break. This helps him to stay on track and to save a bit of money. He may even find time to squeeze a cheeky siesta in between his first meal and going to work. And we all know how glorious a little post-feast snooze can be. Later on in the evening, being able to eat during his break at work makes Mo happy. By shifting his feeding window to close at eleven, he can have his last meal during this break. Perhaps he could even accommodate for a cheeky whisky in there too, which makes dealing with drunk and rowdy tourists a little less taxing. If Mo finishes eating at eleven and starts again at three the next day, then he is still fasting for sixteen hours. The only difference is that these times are much more convenient for his lifestyle. This kind of timeframe serves to *enhance* his lifestyle rather than hinder it, and that is the goal of a fasting lifestyle.

In time, Mo can establish a natural rhythm of fasting and feeding perfectly in sync with his lifestyle. On a typical day, Mo does not break his fast until he has been to the gym and completed any outstanding errands. Some days, this could mean breaking fast at three on the dot, whereas on others it could mean twenty-five past two or four p.m. These minor differences in timings are inconsequential. The important thing is that Mo is exercising flexibility and making fasting into a *lifestyle* rather than a chore.

The key is to find your groove and aim to tie the pattern of fasting and feeding to regular events rather than specific times. This means the clock will not catch us staring at it, and the whole process becomes rather effortless and enjoyable. Another benefit of this flexible approach is that Mo can mix it up on any occasion that life may request it of him. Some days he might be busy with a long list of errands, and to save time, he could elect to fast for longer than usual. Some days, he may have a big lunch with friends on the cards, or perhaps he just wants to eat a little more, so he can extend his feeding window. Some days, he may not even fast at all, whereas other days he may do a prolonged fast and just go without eating right through the whole day. The key is flexibility. Remember, your lifestyle comes first, and we should use fasting as a tool to enhance our lifestyle.

RIDING THE HUNGER WAVE

Hunger is a genetic signal that reminds us to find food. During the time of Zug, in which food was scarce, hunger was the motivation to find dinner. However, today we have food in abundance, so we must be mindful of how often we entertain this signal.

Hunger is like a wave, and it usually subsides after half an hour. But what should we do when this wave hits?

The most effective way to ride the wave of hunger is to stay busy. Naturally, I propose making a list. But not just any list. This is a list of things to complete before you eat: a collection of small tasks that will keep you busy until you plan to break the fast. If you are focussed on completing a task, then the hunger waves will not trouble you. Besides, fasting can heighten mental clarity and energy levels, so we may as well make the most of it by getting stuck into the things that need to get done. Remember that Mother Nature designed hunger with motivation in mind. For most of our evolution, it served as a motivation to find food. But now we have food, so we can use this motivation to get things done. It's also important to consider our surroundings. Wherever possible, try not to put yourself in an environment where temptation is high. For example, if I'm idling in the kitchen during a fast, then the hunger will be harder to resist than if I was walking the dog. Avoiding boredom is key. How many people do you know that proclaim to eat out of boredom? Staying busy is the secret to success, and if you find yourself with nothing to do, then just keep moving. Keeping busy is how we beat hunger at its own game. It makes fasting easier, but it will also benefit other areas of life. By staying busy, we can increase our NEAT, get more done, and enhance our enjoyment of each waking day. The next helping hand is slightly different, coming in the form of *cinnamon*.

I have always enjoyed my coffee black, with no extras. Even before the days of fasting, I was never a fan of milk. And definitely not sugar. Sweet enough darling. I'm a big fan of the taste, so black coffee is a pleasure for me. Many people I meet, however, do not share this attitude, and they often struggle to have their coffee black during a fast. This is where cinnamon can come in. Adding a sprinkle of cinnamon to your coffee is a great way to keep the taste buds engaged and knock out any cravings that may arise during a fast. Scientific research also thinks highly of cinnamon, suggesting that it can improve insulin sensitivity and reduce inflammation[*]. More importantly, cinnamon is delicious and arguably the best natural sweetener out there. In terms of practical application, allow me to share with you my cinnamon

---

[*]which is effectively enhancing the beneficial effects of fasting.

coffee *master tip*. This will work best with a coffee machine that uses capsules. Rather than applying it as a sprinkle on top, what I like to do is stir it in as I, or the machine, pour the coffee. This infuses more of the flavour and creates a cremè-like layer on top, adding texture and body.

Sparkling water is one of the best beverages for keeping the hunger waves at bay. Trust me on this one. Before I discovered fasting, I was never a fan of sparkling water. In fact, I thought it was disgusting, but now I am hooked. In one study from the St. Marianna University School of Medicine in Japan, a group of women fasted overnight before drinking either still or sparkling water. The women who drank the sparkling water scored much higher on a fullness scale compared to those who drank the still water, even though they had eaten nothing. Sparkling water is satisfying and more interesting than plain water. If you don't like it now, you will love it soon enough.

That's a promise.

Hunger is like a **wave**.

It doesn't last for very long, and the more accustomed you become to fasting, the smoother you will negotiate these waves.

BREAKING THE FAST

Most people waste their entire life in a perpetual state of emotional
exhaustion, worrying about things that are beyond their control.
The irony of worrying about things you can't control is that because
they affect your emotions, they control you instead.

- ED LATIMORE

'Will a slice of lemon break the fast?'

'Will chewing gum break the fast?'

'Will inhaling the lovely scent from my new vanilla candle break the fast?'

Let's calm down for a moment. There are far too many people getting hung up on minor details that will ultimately prove inconsequential.

In the discussion of what breaks a fast, opinions will vary. But remember, there are people out there who want to complicate things and create confusion, so they can sell you things you do not need. Fasting is simple, and I advise you to steer clear of anyone who says otherwise. Some people are so quick to say whether something breaks the fast, that they forget to clarify what *breaking the fast* means. Therefore, we must define it. And to do that, we must clarify our *purpose* for fasting.

I fast to simplify life, to control the energy balance, and to enhance the enjoyment of both food and everyday life. So, will something minor like a slice of lemon break the purpose of my fast? No. Likewise, getting caught up in all these complications *will* break the purpose, which is why I like to keep fasting as *simple* as possible.

Whether something breaks the fast is context dependent. So you must clarify your context. The best approach will always be the simple one. Stick to water, black coffee, and green tea during the fasting period.

On a physiological level, many regard insulin as the key factor in deciding whether something breaks the fast. Because when we raise insulin, the body leaves the fat-burning state. Therefore, many people will say that if something raises insulin, it breaks the fast. Dietary fat does not elicit an insulin response, which has led many to conclude that certain items are acceptable to consume during a fast. For example, MCT oil* contains calories, but it derives them from fat. Therefore, consuming MCT oil during a fast will not raise insulin levels, and will keep the body in a fat-burning state. The difference being that the body is now burning dietary fat from an *external* source as opposed to the body fat we have in storage.

When we consider these elements and attempt to juggle them all, everything gets a little too complicated for my liking. For me, fasting means staying away from calories, regardless of what form they come in. Water, black coffee, and green tea keeps it simple. Fasting can simplify your life, but you must allow it to do so.

People often ask me whether chewing gum is acceptable when fasting. And I say *yes*. Researchers from the Tokyo Medical and Dental University found that chewing gum helps to control appetite and impulsive eating behaviour. Chewing gum also freshens your breath, which is a welcome addition during a fast. But make sure there is no sugar involved.

Most people view the transition between the fasted and fed state

---

* MCT oil is a supplement made from a type of fat called medium-chain triglycerides. It is usually made from coconut oil.

similar to flicking a light switch. For example, they think if they accidentally add a splash of milk into their coffee, they have flicked the switch to leave the fasted state. And they have now wasted the time they spent fasting. Not only are they being hard on themselves, the concept itself does not make sense.

Rather than view the transition between the fasted state and the fed state as a switch, a superior approach is to view it as a *dimmer*. A splash of milk will nudge the dimmer up slightly, but we will slide back down to the fasted state after we metabolise this energy. A large meal, however, will turn the dimmer up to the tune of ten to twelve hours.

What you can consume during a fast is all about minimising risk. Water is essential, and black coffee and green tea are low-risk items. They don't seem to interrupt the fast on a physiological level, and they can be great aids to remain consistent with fasting. However, if we take something like diet drinks with artificial sweeteners, we increase the risk. There is still some debate surrounding how they interact with the body on a physiological level while in the fasted state. But they may also open something of a dangerous door. For example, if I'm to consume a diet drink, it stimulates my appetite and I crave more of that sweet taste. I become distracted, and the fast becomes somewhat challenging. And for what? A few moments of mouth pleasure? Not worth the risk. Keep things simple instead.

One of the main reasons I like to promote simple fasting is that it leads us to drink more water. And water is amazing. The vast majority of people will drink more water with fasting in their lifestyle, and we should not overlook this benefit.

The Nutrition Information Center in New York found that 75 percent of Americans are dehydrated. Dehydration is stressful. It can cause fatigue, it clouds memory, and it makes concentrating a challenge. Fasting can combat dehydration. Realistically, it is difficult *not* to drink more water during the fasting period. And it can also form positive habit loops surrounding water intake. For example, if we train ourselves to drink more water, the next time we feel thirsty, we will choose water over a soft drink. And we are better off for it. There is no bigger waste of calories than those in liquid form. Studies have shown that increasing water intake can prevent headaches, increase feelings of wellbeing and improve exercise performance. One study from Virginia Tech found that participants who drank more water during a dieting phase ended up eating less on average. Drinking water is essential for creating a healthy lifestyle. And fasting makes it easier to drink more water.

Fasting reduces decision fatigue. If we are worrying about whether something breaks the fast, we are accumulating decision fatigue and subtracting from other areas of life. On a physiological level, whether anything outside water, black coffee, and green tea will break the fast is still up for debate, so why risk it? A simple approach is the most logical one. By entertaining other decisions, we are allowing ourselves more opportunity for a headache. Besides, fasting itself is much easier when we keep it clean. Embrace the simplicity. That's the beauty of fasting.

I can't drink coffee without heavy cream.

- KATIE GOLDBRIDGE
2018

Katie wanted to incorporate fasting into her life, but she was *adamant* that she could not drink black coffee. My response was blunt, but justifiably so. I told her that she was wrong.

There is plenty of negativity in the world. We face it daily. But sometimes, we are the architects of our own downfall because we tell ourselves we cannot do something. I used to think I could never ride a bicycle. But to achieve anything, we must first at least try. I told Katie to forget about all the nuanced details and the science and to give black coffee a go. I assured her that if she could conquer this small feat, it would be a *game-changer*. She came back a month later and said she was enjoying her coffee without the cream. She had unleashed her inner Italian and was now all about that short espresso lifestyle.

'It's crazy how I was so convinced I needed cream. I can't believe I placed such limitations on myself.'

She is probably liberating herself from other self-imposed limitations as we speak. To break down a barrier is empowering, and it starts with the small ones.

My advice is to keep it as simple as possible. Free yourself from all the dependencies and nonsense, and stick to water, black coffee, and green tea. Likewise, if you accidentally splash some cream in your morning coffee, don't panic. We are aiming for consistency. Not perfection.

Don't lose sight of the big picture by getting caught up in the minor details.

TIME TO EAT

Now the fasting period is complete, and it is time to break the fast. How should you go about it?

There will be some occasions when you have little choice in how you break your fast. On other occasions you *will* have choices. Here are some tips to make some good ones.

- Remember the digestive system has been taking a break, so avoid introducing too much food too soon, as it can cause discomfort and bloating.

- If the situation is not ideal for whatever reason, remember that continuing the fast is always an option. Don't feel you *need* to eat because you've reached a certain point in clock time. For example, you might have been planning to break your fast after sixteen hours.

But when that time arrives, you find yourself in the airport with few options available. Rather than eating for the sake of adhering to a certain timeframe, you can fast for a little longer until there's something better on the table.

It's always an option.

- It is all too tempting to march into the kitchen when it's time to break the fast and eat everything in sight.

Before you know it, you're sitting in your underwear covered in Cheeto dust wondering to yourself *'what just happened?'*

...or perhaps that's just me.

Either way, mistakes can happen without a standard of control in place. To combat this, plan your first meal in advance, and do not allow yourself to stray from this arrangement. You can prepare this meal beforehand, but the important thing is to know what you will eat and stick to it.

- In the first meal, prioritise *protein*. Foods high in protein are satisfying, which will help to keep your appetite under control. Many people struggle to consume enough protein during their feeding window, so getting a good amount in right away is a good strategy. Avoid sugar and anything easy to over-consume.

Short-term fasting should be *simple*. It does not have to be a meticulous operation. However, longer-term fasting of twenty-four hours and upwards is a different matter. When fasting for longer periods of time, it is important to keep the fast clean and to break it with care. But that is a topic that we shall break down in depth in part four.

FASTING AND FITNESS

Physical fitness is not only one of the most important keys to a healthy body, it is the basis of dynamic and creative intellectual activity.

JOHN F. KENNEDY

Conventional wisdom suggests that exercising in the fasted state is a bad idea. But I believe it is an authentic pattern of human behaviour. You will echo this belief soon. And if you don't, the drinks are on me.

The prevalent view is that we *must* eat before exercise, because if we do not, we will not have energy. This assumption, however, stems from a very antiquated school of thought. The people who think like this are still driving in the slow lane, as they have neglected to consider one factor that changes everything. When we enter the fasted state, we still have access to *plenty* of energy; it just comes from stored fat rather than an external food source.

The notion we need to eat before exercise to supply us with sufficient energy is a fallacy. We need not eat food for energy before exercise. One day you will see me shouting this from a rooftop. Don't forget to wave.

Eating has never made me feel energetic. In fact, it has always had the *opposite* effect on me. After a big meal, the last thing I want to do is get my running shoes on. Having to eat before exercise to have sufficient energy is a concept that seems nonsensical to me now. And when we look at it from an evolutionary perspective, this popular notion falls apart even further. The food supply that we enjoy today only represents a blink of the eye in terms of human evolution. If we imagine the human story on earth as a book, then modern food availability would only appear on the last page. Hunting, gathering, and periods of food scarcity, however, would be a regular fixture on several hundred of the previous pages. Humans have been hunting, gathering, and exercising in the fasted state since time began because they had little choice in the matter. It was a question of *survival*. If humans could not rely on their physical capabilities in the fasted state, then they would not have been able to survive the frequent periods of food scarcity.

We need not eat for energy before exercise. It makes little sense. Don't let the bone head personal trainers fool you with their obsolete claims.

To shed light on the subject, researchers from the University of Limerick in Ireland reviewed forty-six studies involving fasted and fed state exercise. They found that fasting did not have a negative impact on performance. Exercising on an empty stomach is possible. But is it *optimal?*

Studies have shown that burning fat for fuel during exercise can increase endurance. The more metabolically flexible we are, the more energy we have access to, and the longer we can exercise. Fasting increases metabolic flexibility, as we are depleting glucose and tapping into fat for fuel. If you are comfortable in the fasted state, there will be no problem with exercise. It may even *benefit* your performance. According to the biomedical scientist Karen Van Proeyen, who is also an exercise expert and long-distance runner herself:

Regular fasted training is a useful strategy to stimulate physiological adaptations in muscle that may eventually contribute to improve endurance exercise performance.

But real life is not so simple. And personal preference always plays a part. I love to exercise in the fasted state. It feels natural to me. But others will not feel the same way. Even before fasting, it always felt right to go running on an empty stomach. When I play football*, I find my performance improves if I'm deep into the fasted state. I always like to be between twenty and twenty-four hours fasted to play sports. And I call this the *primal power zone*. Optimal performance is a subjective matter. Try it for yourself and see.

Human beings are resilient. We are the descendants of those who could exert themselves physically while in the fasted state. And the fact of the matter is we can achieve great things without food in our belly. Being active and exercising to a high level on an empty stomach is an authentic pattern of human behaviour. I believe that an empty stomach is the natural human state for exercise. As for energy, the body already has plenty. It's called *fat*. When we fast, we use fat for fuel. When we exercise while fasting, we use even more. So how does fasted exercise interact with fat loss?

As we discussed earlier, fat burn does not always equate to fat loss. The fundamentals of the energy balance still apply. But increasing the amount of fat we burn will be of great help in managing the energy balance. This is because we are burning *more* energy, so we increase the amount of energy out in the energy balance equation, which gives us a lot more calorie freedom. Scientists have linked fat burning to a higher rate of success in losing weight and keeping it off in various studies. But we shall dive into that topic in greater detail in chapter five.

The bottom line: You do not need to eat before exercise. Perhaps exercising on an empty stomach is natural. Try it for yourself.

MUSCLE

Barry at the gym will probably tell you that fasting and building muscle are not compatible. And for a long time, I echoed this viewpoint.

I subscribed to the broscience; I bought all the supplements, and

---

*which is ninety minutes of intense running if the manager does not leave me on the bench (unfortunately, this happens often)

I associated fasting with a lack of strength. But upon reflection, I was wrong. Before we dive in, let's clear something up. Fasting will *not* burn muscle. This is the overwhelming consensus, but it is not a science-based view. First, fasting increases growth hormone production, which directly operates to maintain muscle mass. Fasting is muscle-*sparing*. Not muscle-burning. But more on that in the next part. If we consult the data, there is nothing to suggest that intermittent fasting has any negative impact on muscle mass. In fact, quite the opposite. One study that was published in the *Journal of Translational Medicine* in 2016 found that people who used intermittent fasting during a dieting phase maintained *more* muscle mass than those who did not use fasting. If you incorporate fasting into your lifestyle, you will not be at a disadvantage in terms of performance in the gym or building muscle. If fasting burned muscle, we would not be here today. It is that simple.

With or without fasting, building muscle is tough. In fact, I would even say that building muscle is harder than losing fat. Building and maintaining muscle mass is a marathon. It requires equal parts dedication, hard work, and patience. First, let's talk about the basics.

Nutrition matters in muscle growth. But some people make it more complicated than it is. Bodybuilding wisdom has made the directive rather clear. You need to eat big to get big. And this may be one of the few fragments of conventional wisdom that holds some truth, though it has been wildly exaggerated. According to the data, it is necessary to eat in a calorie surplus to stimulate muscle growth. This means that we need to consume more energy than the body requires. If we are eating more than we need, this means that fat loss will be off the table while building muscle is the goal. Although some studies have shown people building muscle and losing fat at the same time, it is quite rare. And usually only seen in people who are overweight or have very low levels of muscle mass to begin with. It is just a lot more straightforward to stimulate muscle growth if we have excess energy. Just imagine that you are building a house. If you have more supplies available, building the structure becomes a lot easier and less stressful.

However, consuming more calories is not the only factor in muscle growth. We also need to consider how much protein we are consuming. Protein plays a crucial role in muscle growth because it stimulates muscle protein synthesis. This is the body repairing and rebuilding the muscle tissue that we broke down in the gym, so it can grow back bigger and stronger. This may come as a shock to some people, as they believe that their muscles are growing while they are working out in the gym, but the opposite is true. When we lift weights, we are putting the muscles under stress and breaking them down, which is why it is important to allow them to recover. Training is just one piece of the puzzle. We also require adequate nutrition and recovery for our muscles to grow.

Exactly how much protein we should consume has generated a fair amount of debate over the years. In bodybuilding folklore, the typical *bro* answer is to aim for one gram of protein per pound of body weight, or 2.2 grams per kilo of bodyweight. However, measuring protein intake according to total body weight is a flawed approach. According to this heuristic, a 250lb person with very high levels of body fat would aim to consume 250 grams of protein a day. This is not only very difficult to do, but also unnecessary for their body composition. A better way to approach the question would be to take the same equation but measure protein intake according to *lean body mass*, which is body weight minus body fat. For example, my total body weight is 210 pounds/95 kilograms, and I'm sitting at around 10 percent body fat. I can roughly estimate that my lean body mass will be around 189 pounds/85.5 kilograms, and that would leave me with a target of 190 grams of protein per day. Even this seems like a high figure, and I have been building muscle with less, but it is not a bad target to aim for. And that's my whole point. As long as we are aiming high regarding our protein intake, it will usually be enough. It is not worth getting too hung up on the numbers unless we are planning to take the pursuit of bodybuilding to a competitive or professional level. My personal advice, though it is not a rigorous measurement by any stretch of the imagination, is to prioritise protein in your nutrition. Make it a priority. And just try to eat a lot. That's it. I have spent many years of my life meticulously tracking my protein intake and worrying if I was eating enough. Now, I just make it a priority in my meals. And given how I've still been able to make progress without worrying about the minor details, it seems to serve me well.

If protein is important, the question is, will you be able to eat enough? Some people struggle to eat enough for muscle growth when they have a small window in which to eat. If this is an issue, just extend the feeding window. The vast majority of people will find that incorporating fasting while focusing on muscle growth allows them to consume enough but not go overboard. Incorporating fasting is the perfect way to carry out a *lean bulk*, which comprises putting on muscle mass without the added fluff*.

Then we come to the next pillar of muscle growth, which is *training*. Many people are unsure whether to train in the fasted state or the fed state. But it makes little difference. Personally, I prefer fasted training. My most explosive sessions come in the *primal power zone†*. But everyone will be different. The most important factor is to find your preference. The pursuit of building muscle is a long journey, so it's important to enjoy the process of training. In my case, fasted state training is superior in terms of muscle growth because I enjoy it and it is something I can maintain for the long run. Building muscle takes time, so find the approach that feels most sustainable for you.

---

*'But I'm bulking, bro' is a common excuse for gym-goers to overindulge.
† Remember me when this phrase goes global.

Training for muscle growth is simple. It's not easy. But it *is* simple. What we need to focus on is progressive overload. And an easy way to explain progressive overload is with the story of Milo of Croton.

Milo was an ancient Greek athlete and renowned wrestler. He began his quest to get big by carrying around a baby calf every day. As the calf grew, so did Milo. The calf grew heavier until it was a fully grown bull, which increased Milo's muscle mass and strength.

As our discussions so far in this book have made clear, the body can adapt to a broad range of challenges. We have seen how it can adapt to the amount of energy we consume and to fasting. But it can also adapt to the demands of resistance training. To continue making gains, we must progressively increase the stress to our muscles as they become stronger. Think like Milo and his growing baby bull. If we do not apply progressive overload to our training, we will eventually hit a plateau and the gain train will come crashing to a halt. There are two main methods to overload the muscle. We can increase the *resistance* by using more weight in our exercises, or we can increase the training *volume* by doing more repetitions, sets, or exercises. The optimal approach is often a mixture of the two. Not that I will have to increase the training volume until I'm doing hundreds of sets and spending hours in the gym, but it is an alternation. For example, one week I might be bicep curling with 12 kg dumbbells for 10 reps. The next week, I will go up to 12 reps. And the week after that I can increase the resistance to 14 kg, but then shift back down to the range of 10 reps*. Another tool in the overload box is to increase the *intensity* of the workout. This means reducing the amount of rest time between sets. Use a mixture of all three to keep your training fresh ensure progress. Over-training is when the body becomes fatigued from too much stress. To avoid it, the American College of Sports Medicine recommend that we change resistance and training volume

---

*This is just an example. I wouldn't make progress this quickly.

in increments of between 2.5% and 5% per week. Remember, it is a long game, slow and steady wins the race.

Keep a training log and plan your workouts ahead of time. Trust me. This will be the best thing you ever do regarding building muscle. Not only does it make it easier to stay motivated, but it is also an efficient method of tracking progress. When making plans, think *big*. When making progress, think *small*. Focus on making the gradual increases over time, and the gains will come.

Moving on to the subject of planning nutrition around training. Let's say that you train in the fasted state. When should you be aiming to break your fast? The common answer is that we should eat as soon as we finish training. And although many swear by their immediate post-workout protein shake, it is perhaps not as important as previously thought. In the bodybuilding world, there was a popular concept known as the anabolic window*. Everyone believed they had to eat within this anabolic window to maximise their gains. This idea is perhaps the reason so many people feel the need to consume protein as soon as they finish working out, and panic if they cannot do so. But they have misplaced their worries. A comprehensive review published in the *Journal of the International Society of Sports Nutrition* shed light on the validity of the anabolic window. Researchers found that this window does not exist. They concluded that the most important factor in muscle growth is the *total* nutrient intake, regardless of the timing. The research suggests that eating sooner rather than later following a training session is optimal for muscle growth. But unless someone is taking bodybuilding to a competitive or professional level, I would not worry about it. Aim to break your fast soon after training, but don't worry if you can't.

Now that we've spent a bit of time together, there is something I

---

*The anabolic window was a concept in which many believed that protein *had* to be consumed in the hour following a workout, or they would not make gains.

must confess. Not so long ago, supplements had me in shackles. And the realisation that it was a problem only dawned on me when I was flying from Barcelona to London with two huge suitcases in tow.

You know how it is. Packing a suitcase is always a stressful affair. Not only do you have to worry if you have remembered everything. But also to make sure it stays below a certain weight or risk being charged an astronomical fee. When I reached the check-in desk, the beautiful lady on the other side welcomed me with a warm smile. As I tossed my first case onto the scale, her smile turned into a frown. She looked at me as if I had deeply wronged her, and informed me I was ten kilos overweight. She presented me with a choice: I could either pay the extra charge. Or check in another bag, which was a considerably cheaper option. Fortunately, I am no stranger to females losing their patience with me, so I could keep a cool head. I had planned for this scenario and had packed an extra bag, so I could check that in and avoid the outrageous fees.

As I unzipped my heavier suitcase to extract the spare bag, the two hundred passengers queuing behind me watched on as a white haze rose from inside my luggage. While I was dragging these massive suitcases around the city like a madman, my supplement containers must have broken because of the turbulence. As a result, a fine white powder had infiltrated every nook and cranny of my suitcase. And now it was all over my face too. It would amuse to add that I was sweaty and dishevelled after all the travelling and getting flummoxed at the desk, which amplified my already suspicious appearance. To my pleasant surprise, the police did not wrestle me from my luggage and whisk me away for questioning. I got the job done and passed through security. I even had enough time to dust myself off before boarding the plane, so as not to appear like a powdered puff pastry for the entire flight.

Everything worked out okay, but it was still a transformative experience.

In the days that followed, I subjected myself to some rigorous questioning. Do I need all these supplements? Are they worth the money? Eventually, I had to accept the fact that I had fallen into the trap of blindly believing the marketing hype. In doing so, I neglected to do my research. It was time to relax a little and liberate myself from this dependence on supplements.

Fast forward to the present day, and I am in the best shape of my life. I'm lean, strong, and I feel good. I have used no muscle building or fat loss supplements for several years now. Not even protein powder. Instead, I've been focusing on the fundamental principles of training, nutrition and recovery. And it has brought the best results to date.

Let's be clear, some supplements *can* be beneficial for certain people. Protein powder can be useful. If someone struggles to eat enough protein, then supplementing with it is an easy solution. But it is just an additional source of protein. Nothing more. It does not have any magical muscle building properties. And it is *not* essential.

People often ask me if taking a BCAA (Branched-Chain Amino Acids) supplement will break the fast. But perhaps they are asking the wrong question. They should instead ask *why* they are taking it.

Many people seem to think supplementing with BCAAs is necessary, but this is not the case. First, some people believe that supplementing with BCAAs during a fasting period prevents the breakdown of muscle. But as we have discussed already, fasting does not burn muscle; rather, it is muscle-sparing, so this should not be a concern. That is the first conundrum easily solved. The second is the prevalent belief that supplementing with BCAAs is necessary for muscle growth. There are many influential figures in the fitness industry who echo this claim, but there is no scientific evidence to support it. Before we get into that, let's talk about amino acids.

BCAAs make up three of the nine essential amino acids* (EAA) that the body requires for building new muscle tissue. They are essential in the sense that the body can not produce them and therefore we need to take them in through our diet. It is important to understand that stimulating muscle protein synthesis, which is building new muscle, requires the availability of *all* the EAAs. Not *just* the BCAAs. So supplementation of BCAAs alone will not support an increased rate of muscle growth. All high-quality protein sources, like the humble egg for example, contain the full range of EAAs, including the three BCAAs. Therefore, if a person is already consuming a sufficient amount of high-quality protein, then they will already stimulate muscle protein synthesis. And additional BCAA supplementation will offer no benefit. If we are already consuming a decent amount of protein, which we should aim to do anyway, then supplementing with BCAAs will be pointless. Like turning the sprinkler on when it's already raining. As sports scientist Robert R. Wolfe concluded in his review of the subject:

The claim that consumption of dietary BCAAs stimulates muscle protein synthesis or produces an anabolic response in human subjects is unwarranted.

Don't worry about BCAA's. Just get the protein. Although those who can profit from endorsing it support the purported efficacy of BCAA supplementation, the research does not. Don't trust the juiced-up social media starlets. They are after your money. With BCAA's, the marketing giant has very much overshadowed the scientific evidence. In summary, instead of BCAAs, I recommend a combination of SPI (sufficient protein intake). CT (consistent training). POS (plenty of sleep). And a healthy dose of SYM (saving your money). Don't worry about BCAAs. Stay on top of your protein intake and the

---

*The three BCAAs are leucine, isoleucine and valine. The other six EAAs are tryptophan, histidine, threonine, phenylalanine, methionine and lysine.

gains will come. While we are on the subject, research has shown that two other supplements that I used to swear by, L-Glutamine and CLA, are more or less *useless*. Going direct to scientific research, rather than trust fitness personalities and magazines, has saved me a lot of cash. Although I wasted money on many supplements, I was never a fan of pre-workout. It always made my head itch. Some people ask me if it breaks the fast, and I say they should avoid it. Why? Because it's just an expensive hit of caffeine. Get that black coffee in your system instead, and skip the itchy head. Don't forget the fact that fitness supplements are part of a multi-million dollar industry. And many influential figures in the fitness space have made a lot of money by endorsing them. Therefore, it is important to do our research. We cannot trust the word of the salesman. Although a lot of these influential fitness figures credit supplements for their physique, they are usually unnaturally enhanced. Supplements had nothing to do with their physique. It is just a pack of lies to sell more piffle. The whole thing is a facade. It's a disgrace. Especially with so many impressionable young people using social media.

Supplements: we do not need them. The best supplement is a good night's sleep. And it always will be. So save your shillings and invest that money into a nice bouquet for your mother instead. Oh, and while we're on the subject, please, do not even *consider* going near fat-burning supplements or anyone who is trying to peddle them. The only thing they will burn is your money. The ultimate fat-burning supplement is free. It's *fasting*.

Can you build muscle with intermittent fasting? Yes. Of course you can. In building muscle, it is the fundamentals that are key. Whether someone fasts makes little difference. If you can master the basic principles of training, nutrition and recovery, then you can build muscle even if you fast for twenty-three hours of the twenty-four in a day.

~~WHEN~~
WHAT TO EAT

It is the mark of a charlatan to explain a simple concept

in a complex way.

- NAVAL RAVIKANT

I love talking about when to eat. I could talk about it all day.
But how about *what* to eat?

If you are looking for specific guidance regarding nutrition, I apologise in advance. I rarely get involved in the discussion of what to eat, and when I do, I stick to basic principles. Tackling the question of what to eat is tricky, and there are several variables at play. Allergies, tastes, intolerances, preferences and budget, to name a few.

In nutrition, there is no black and white; rather, it is all shades of grey. However, there are a few principles that we can all agree on. One effective step that anyone can take that will get them leaner and healthier is to avoid ultra-processed foods. As a study from the National Institutes of Health showed, sticking to unprocessed foods naturally regulates our appetite, which often results in effortless calorie control. Another wise strategy is to avoid soft drinks and liquid calories. It is always more satisfying to *eat* calories rather than drink them.

Nutrition is fascinating. However, the Internet is a misleading place, and there are many charlatans over-complicating it. The fact is that there will never be one approach that suits everyone.

Eating is not just digestion; there is a multitude of other processes taking place. The absorption and distribution of nutrients, their uptake by receptors, their transport across cells, their storage, and finally, their excretion. Consider how complex the biochemical makeup of each human is, and how much variability there is between every one of us. With all that in mind, how likely is it we will react to certain foods in the same way? When I was a child, I convinced myself that I was allergic to vegetables. As I got older, I forced myself to eat them, and now I rather enjoy them. We can train our tastes, but we have less control over how our bodies react to certain foods.

Figuring out a way of eating that works for you while aligning with your goals and lifestyle is not easy, and it will require patience. The key principle is to understand that the energy balance governs weight loss, maintenance, and gain. How we react to certain foods depends on several variable factors, but we know that the concept of the energy balance applies across the board. To gain a deeper understanding of the energy balance, we must consider where calories come into the equation. Calories measure *energy*. Everything in the body utilises energy, and we need to consume it to sustain life. When we fast, we break down stored fat to release energy. Likewise, when we eat food, we break it down into energy which, depending on the energetic requirements of the body, is utilised immediately or stored for later use. Some say that calories do not matter, but to totally disregard them would be a flawed approach. Much like weight or distance, calories are just a measurement. Are ten kilograms of feathers the same as ten kilograms of granite? They are different in many ways, but they *weigh* the same. Two people weigh 95 kilograms. One has a significant amount of well developed lean muscle mass with low levels of body fat, and the other has minimal muscle mass with high levels of body fat. They are on opposite ends of the body composition spectrum, but they *weigh* the same. Running a mile on the beach is harder than running a mile on the Olympic track, but it's still a mile. There is no need to demonise calories nor exile them. They are just a measurement and we can use them as a rough guideline. Obsessing over calories and prioritising them over everything else is a flawed approach, but they can be a useful tool to add to our box. Nutrition is confusing, but understanding calories and the energy balance is *empowering* and allows a person to make progress while they fine-tune the more intricate details of their nutrition.

Some people say that calories don't matter after incorporating fasting. Many enjoy great results with fasting without thinking about calories, feeding the misconception that fasting is magical and allows us to eat whatever we want and still get results. What these people may not realise is that they are still restricting their energy intake. The difference is that they are not putting in effort to do so, as opposed to a person who is tracking all of their calorie intake. Fasting facilitates *effortless* calorie control. But it's still calorie control. When some people say you need not restrict calories following incorporating fasting, perhaps what they mean is that you need not pay calories much attention. Fasting creates an environment in which maintaining an energy deficit is effortless. In the discussion of sustainable fat loss, we often confuse the terms *restrict* and *count*. When someone says that you need not restrict calories, what they often mean to say is that you need not attempt to count calories.

That leaves us with one question. Should you count calories?

Well, you might not *need* to. Fasting makes managing the energy balance effortless. Many people find that after incorporating fasting, they see results without changing their nutrition or tracking their calorie intake, but the fundamentals still apply. Understanding energy balance does not have to be a chore; rather, it can be quite empowering. If you have implemented some kind of fasting and have observed no progress, or hit a plateau, then consider grabbing calories by the scruff of the neck and taking control. But before you do so, I want you to make sure you are living as close to authentic patterns of human behaviour as possible. Before you consider counting calories, ask yourself the following questions.

Am I drinking calories? I am a firm believer that liquid calories are a waste of time. They are not satisfying, and can quickly add up and drag fat loss to a halt. Stick to water.

Am I prioritising my sleep? Sleeping more will not directly lead to an increased rate of fat loss, but it can positively influence several behaviors that will. Aim for eight hours a night and a consistent bedtime.

Am I attempting to be as active as possible? You don't have to run yourself into the ground with excessive exercise. But making small changes to your daily life to become more active can make a world of difference. We shall go over this concept with a fine-tooth comb in part six.

Am I gravitating to whole food choices? I don't believe that we have to complicate nutrition, but highly processed foods are often calorie dense and easy to over-consume. Avoid them when possible.

Am I prioritising protein? For many people, eating more protein can be a game changer because of its satiating nature. Healthy protein intake keeps your appetite in check. Don't skimp on it.

Am I letting myself go on weekends? Staying on track during the week is rather straightforward when there are few distractions. However, when the weekend arrives and the festivities begin, it can get a little harder. Those drinks have calories too, remember. And a hangover can disrupt even the best-laid plans for a healthy lifestyle. Don't deprive yourself of fun, but don't forget the importance of balance either.

Estimating calorie intake, unless you have prior experience of tracking calories, is not the best idea. I can estimate my calorie intake with a fair accuracy, but I have spent a lot of time rigorously tracking my calorie intake in the past. Tracking calories indefinitely is not a sustainable approach, nor is it required. It feels very robotic, and it made me feel miserable after a while. Chances are, it will make *you* feel miserable too. Tracking calories for a short time, however, can be an eye-opener, and bring clarity to the process. For further clarification, let's check in with some old friends.

Mo is making progress, but his partner Julia has hit a *plateau*. She toys with various ideas to get her journey going again. Perhaps giving up wine is the answer? Maybe she should stay an extra half an hour in the gym? or cut out carbohydrates? These measures *could* work, but it is a stab in the dark. A rather hit and hope approach, if you will. I propose a two-week plan to Julia that could add clarity, change the way she views the journey, and empower her. For two weeks, Julia will track all of her calorie intake with the help of an app*.

Julia tracks everything for the next two weeks. It's a hassle at first, but after a few days it becomes much easier. At the end, she had made two observations that will be invaluable for creating a healthy lifestyle. First, she was unaware that she was consuming such a large amount of calories from things that offered her little to no satisfaction. For example, the juice that she drinks at work contains a significant amount of calories, but it offers her no satisfaction. She can swap it out for water at no cost to her quality of life equation but of huge benefit to her progress. By doing so, she can alter her *lifestyle*, rather than implement a quick fix or drastic measure. If a change is not sustainable, it's not worth it. The second observation is that after two weeks, nothing had changed. Her body composition, weight, and measurements were all the same. This is not a bad thing; in fact, it's what we were looking for. Because she has maintained her weight, she now knows roughly what her *maintenance* level of energy intake is, which is the amount she needs to consume to maintain her weight. It is not an exact measurement by any stretch of the imagination, but it's

---

*My personal recommendation would be MyFitnessPal.

a helpful figure. Shaving a few calories off that amount, by taking the juice out her life for example, or by walking to work instead of taking the bus, could get her progress going again.

It will not be the most riveting fortnight in the world, but it *will* be an empowering one. Fat loss requires energy restriction, be it through reducing intake or increasing output. When we have a clear picture of where our intake comes from, we replace the ambiguity with *clarity*. This makes it easier to implement sustainable changes, as opposed to relying on drastic measures and enduring the inevitable frustration.

Many people use an online calculator to find out their Total Daily Energy Expenditure (TDEE), which is the average number of calories one will burn in a day. They will take the subsequent calculation as gospel, but there is no way that a simple equation could ever provide you with an accurate number. This misinformation can lead to even more frustration and confusion. Regarding how many calories we burn in a day, there are a multitude of factors at play[*]. Our energy expenditure is not a fixed rate; rather, it is constantly fluctuating. Tracking calorie intake will never be an exact science, but it gives us a rough ballpark figure to work with. Rather than an exact guide, it's a helpful indicator. When considering calorie expenditure, avoid using any online calculator. Julia's method, although it requires a little more effort, is much more effective.

You might find that you need not worry about calories during your journey, but working with them can be helpful. Remember, calorie restriction in some kind of format is necessary for weight loss; it's just a lot easier to do so when we incorporate fasting into our lifestyle.

The details of nutrition will vary wildly and contain many complexities, but the fundamentals are simple.

---

[*]Even the brain uses a significant amount of energy. According to Robert Sapolsky, a Stanford professor of neurology and neurosurgery, a chess grandmaster can burn up to 6,000 calories a day during a tournament. Despite the fact that they are sitting down for most of the time.

FLEXIBILITY

It's more important to do big things well
than to do the small things perfectly.

- RAY DALIO

It's 10 pm on a Friday night and it's been an awfully long week.

You and some close friends have finished dinner with a few exquisite bottles of wine. The consensus of the group is to move on to a bar for cheeky drinks and a shake of the leg. There's just one problem though. You usually close your fasting window at 8 pm, and it's already gone well past that hour. What should you do? You may feel like calling it a night to rush home and bask in the warm glow of discipline before whisking yourself off for an early night, but life is short. Now, you could exercise your best behaviour and resist the temptation to get a little sloshy, and there will be times when this will be the best option. Upon reflection, there are plenty of episodes in my life that I should have called a little earlier. But leaving the festivities prematurely won't be the best option on *every* occasion.

If I was to indulge in every opportunity to go out for drinks, food or a combination of both, then I doubt that I would be very healthy at all. But if I was to *decline* the vast majority of those opportunities because they didn't fit my fasting schedule or fitness regime, then I would be miserable. It is important to be open to these opportunities now and again. Life is defined by spontaneous experiences with the people we love, or perhaps a special person who we may even end up falling in love with.

When we expose the brain to novelty, time slows down. Psychologists refer to this phenomenon as the oddball effect, in which experiencing new stimuli can exaggerate our perception of time. Have you ever noticed how a weekend in a new city always seems to last longer than a weekend spent doing the same old thing? This is the oddball effect in full swing. Conversely, locking oneself into a routine of doing the same thing repeatedly like clockwork will only speed up time, and before you know it another year has passed. To make the most out of life, we must be open to experiencing new things. If not, it will all be over far too soon.

Regarding the incorporation of fasting, we must remind ourselves of our underlying intention. We want a sustainable healthy lifestyle, not a quick fix. Therefore, it is paramount to establish a balance. If we are too strict on ourselves regarding the timeframe of our fasting, then it will likely end in frustration. We need to have some flexibility with fasting, so we can incorporate it successfully as part of a lifestyle rather than just a short-term fling. Long-term success is all about the give and take.

Before I discovered fasting, my destructive dieting habits were a prison. I was always worrying about whether something was healthy, and I resented having to do anything that meant going even slightly off track. And my track was narrow. I spent the vast majority of my time and mental energy focusing on my nutrition and my physique, which began to subtract from my life and those around me.

Was it worth it? Absolutely not. And I'm thankful that I escaped this negative mindset. Things are different now. When an opportunity arises for eating and drinking with family or friends, I can honour it with pleasure rather than passing it up, because I have that fasting flexibility.

Let's use Mo as an example again.

Something rather peculiar has happened to Mo. He has the weekend off from work, and Mo *never* gets the weekend off from work. This means he does something that he hasn't done in a while. He goes out with his friends on a Saturday night. As I'm sure anyone who has worked in hospitality will agree, this is an opportunity that he cannot pass up. However, Mo is worrying about what this will mean for his fasting schedule and the progress that he has made.

There are two closely connected and very important factors that I try to communicate to Mo. The first is that people have been healthy, lost fat and will continue to do so without diligently adhering to a fasting schedule. Therefore, if we take a few days off from fasting, it is not a big deal. Second, it is hard to move *backwards* on progress. I mean *really* hard. Perhaps if you were to take a few weeks off and really go off the rails, then you may start moving in the opposite direction. But within the space of a few days, there is literally only so much damage that you can do. In the vast majority of cases, taking a break is pressing the *pause* button on progress, not rewind. So press pause, enjoy it for what it is, and when it's over hit that play button again with even more vigour and motivation than before.

Mo acknowledges all of this, but he still wants to maintain some kind of rhythm. Fasting makes him feel *good*, and it has made his lifestyle much easier, so we crack on and start discussing the solutions. The proposed dinner destination is his favourite steak restaurant, and he always eats well there. Mo loves to get a big parrillada for the table, which is a traditional Argentine/Uruguayan meal and essentially an enormous platter of grilled meats. He is no stranger to the homemade tiramisu either. There is no holding back in this establishment. They will also drink several bottles of wine and the chances that they will continue the hoopla into the small hours of the morning are high. Rather than cut the festivities short to follow his fasting schedule to the letter, Mo can engineer his schedule so that everything falls into place.

For example, on Saturday, Mo can extend his fasting window so he either breaks his fast at the steak house with his friends or shortly before. This allows him a lot more room to play with for dinner. If he has spent most of the day fasting, then it will be very difficult to massively over consume calories for the day from just one meal. This is what I like to refer to as *calorie freedom*. With fasting, Mo has calorie freedom, which allows him to enjoy his meal without worrying about going overboard. Realistically, because Mo is eating one large meal, there is very little risk of losing control.

Let's say that Mo finishes consuming calories and begins his fasting period at around 3 a.m. The following day, Mo naturally sleeps in, but still wakes up feeling rather rough. Given his delicate and hungover condition, it is tempting to eat immediately. Specifically, with a big delicious pizza from the Italian place downstairs. Mo, however, wants to give himself longer before starting to eat, so he pushes his breakfast back to 7 p.m., which would make 16 hours since he last ate. Now, he has no choice but to get up and get moving. Before he knew about fasting, hangovers were synonymous with eating junk food and lying around thinking about all the things he said the night before, which only made him feel worse. Now, Mo doesn't have the option to eat, so he instead gets active, gets outside, and gets hydrated. All of which are key factors in combatting the symptoms of a hangover. Later on, when Mo arrives home, he feels fresh and is ready to prepare a wholesome and nutritious meal. Mo closes his feeding window at his usual time of 11 p.m. so he can get a good night's sleep and wake up fresh to attack the following day. Now he's back on track with his usual timing, and because he's adhered to some kind of fasting schedule throughout the festivities, he has stayed perfectly on track with his long-term goals.

Not only did he have calorie freedom on Saturday night, but fasting prevented him from making any poor hangover-induced food choices on Sunday. I'm sure you know of how easy it is to succumb to the temptation of hangover food. I suspect that hangovers may even be a significant factor in the business model of various fast food delivery chains. However, when we embrace fasting and use it as a tool, we need not worry about any of that.

SUMMARY

Fasting keeps it *simple*.

Instead of saying No, be like Mo. Exercise flexibility with fasting and manipulate it around your social life.

Alternatively, you *could* have a break. If a break will help you with adherence in the long run, then it will be infinitely more valuable than being strict and missing out. Both are good strategies and we should consider them before turning down the opportunity to enjoy ourselves.

Remember: Flexibility is key.

Consistency is an easier target to hit than perfection, and the prize is far superior.

Part Four

PROLONGED FASTING

A fasting lifestyle typically involves dividing the day
into fasting and feeding.

Prolonged fasting is when we fast for longer
than the entire duration of the day.

To some it may sound bizarre, but in several cultures and religions,
they associate prolonged periods of fasting
with powerful healing.

In this section, we will look at what the research can tell us about it.

SAFETY

To lengthen thy life,
lessen thy meals.
- BENJAMIN FRANKLIN

Before we jump in, I must stress the importance of safety. As with many other things in life, it is important to do your homework and clarify your intentions.

I'm not a doctor myself, and this is *not* medical advice. This is a discussion of interesting research and my own experiences.

Though I will cover it in more detail towards the end of this section, please also refer back to the first section of the last part (p.65) for a reminder of safety regarding fasting. With that said, let's see what the research can tell us about the safety of prolonged fasting.

The True North Health Center (TNHC) is an integrative medical facility in Santa Rosa, California that uses fasting as a dietary intervention. Some patients at True North may fast for a day or two, whereas some may fast for longer, even as long as twelve days. Researchers took data from 768 patient visits to the TNHC and rated any adverse effects from fasting, such as headaches, on a scale of severity from **1** to **5**.

1- Mild

2- Moderate

3- Severe

4- Life-threatening or disabling

5- Death

Before we begin, I know what you're thinking, and the answer is *no*; they did not record a level 5 event. Out of 768 visits, there were just two adverse events recorded which the researchers considered serious. One was a grade 3 dehydration event that occurred after three days of fasting in a 73-year-old male. He made a full recovery and returned to the center. The other was a grade 4 *hyponatremia* event. When sodium levels are extremely low in the blood, it leads to hyponatremia, which is a life-threatening condition. Sodium is an electrolyte, and we shall cover the topic of electrolyte balance in the following pages. This grade 4 event occurred to a 70-year-old male on the *ninth* day of his prolonged fast. In my opinion, this is an abnormally long time to fast for someone that age. Fortunately, he made a full recovery.

Most adverse events that the researchers recorded were mild and known reactions, such as slight headaches and feelings of fatigue. So what can we learn from this? It suggests that, while the responsible use of prolonged fasting is safe, it is not without risk.

Therefore, we must always practice prolonged fasting with care and attention.

I recently spoke with a lady trying to lose weight for her friend's upcoming wedding. Let's call her Ramona. Ramona had just returned home from a stressful semester at university in which she had put on some extra weight. In a panic, she asked me how she could lose this extra weight in time for the wedding. My reply was not what she wanted to hear. I told her that sustainable fat loss takes time and commitment and it hinges on the fundamentals of energy balance. There are many ways to lose weight in the short-term, but these approaches can end up doing more harm than good. Ignoring my initial response, she asked, '*if I fast for X amount of days, I'll lose X amount of weight, right?*'

This worried me. For starters, it's not that simple. There are many factors that affect fat loss, and rarely does it follow a linear pattern. Besides, we should never use prolonged fasting for fat loss alone. This is unwise and irresponsible, as it can lead to the creation of several negative feedback loops. For example, fasting as punishment following a weekend of indulgence or as a form of crash dieting to prepare for a special event, like a wedding. These are not hallmarks of a healthy lifestyle, and we must avoid these patterns of behaviour. If someone desires to fast for several days with the sole intention of losing weight, then forget it. It will *not* be the answer, and it *will* have negative consequences.

We should practise fasting to distance ourselves from destructive habits, not to exacerbate them.

SET AND SETTING

Nature loves courage.

You make the commitment and nature will respond

to that commitment by removing impossible obstacles.

Dream the impossible dream and the world will not grind you under,

it will lift you up. This is the trick.

This is what all these teachers and philosophers who really counted,

who really touched the alchemical gold,

this is what they understood.

This is the shamanic dance in the waterfall.

This is how magic is done.

By hurling yourself into the abyss

and discovering it's a feather bed.

- TERENCE MCKENNA

Similar to the therapeutic use of psychedelic substances, the *set* and *setting* are very important regarding prolonged fasting.

Set refers to the mindset, which is what the person brings to the experience, and the setting refers to the environment in which they experience it. Let's talk a little about preparation. Before someone undertakes a prolonged fast, it is very important that they are familiar with spending time in the fasted state. If someone with no prior experience jumps into a prolonged fast, they will *not* have fun.

Although often overlooked, the setting is a crucial component of any prolonged fast.

When you fast for a whole day or longer, you realise how much time food consumes from the day. Not having to worry about food is empowering, and it unlocks a new dimension of spare time. To capitalise on this freedom, it is imperative to engage ourselves. Otherwise, the wandering mind will flirt with food, and this subtracts from the experience. Whenever I embark on a prolonged fast, I plan it around times in which I know that I will be the most engaged. If I've got a few hectic days in the calendar, then I will often just fast. It makes life a lot easier. I'm more focused in the fasted state, which helps to navigate the hectic days, and a busy schedule keeps my mind off food. Therefore, the fast becomes somewhat effortless.

Another factor to consider about the setting is how to plan around social commitments. If a date with friends or family appears in the calendar, it will be best for all parties to leave the fasting for another day. Although some may applaud you for your commitment if you fast, it will disappoint most. I save prolonged fasting for days when I know social events will be sparse, meaning you will not see me fasting through the entirety of a weekend.

We should use fasting as a tool to *simplify* life, not complicate it.

Prolonged fasting can seem impossible at first, but it's easy. Society has conditioned us to eat every day throughout our lives, so going a whole day without eating is a strange, but empowering, sensation. However, if it's rocky, then make some changes. For example, if rampant hunger risks interfering with your wellbeing, then don't feel you must persist. Just break the fast and try again later. Likewise, if you have a persistent headache or feel unwell, then first assess your electrolyte balance (more on that later), and consider calling time on the fast. Do not sacrifice your wellbeing for the sake of adhering to the original intended duration of the fast. Regarding the timeframe, don't pay too much attention to the specifics of the numbers; they don't hold too much importance.

Life ebbs and flows. Sometimes you will feel great, other times not so great. React accordingly.

The set is also a crucial element. A negative mindset will lead to negative outcomes. If a person bases their rationale for prolonged fasting in negativity, punishing themselves following indulgence for example, then it will lead to a slippery slope. We must avoid using fasting as punishment. Occasionally, progress is slow, but it's *still* progress. The *direction* of our journey is far more important than the speed. Don't sabotage the gradual creation of a work of art by impatiently seeking small immediate gains.

Going to extreme measures to lose weight is like opening Pandora's Box. Once you entertain these destructive concepts, it becomes difficult to control them, and they have no place in any lifestyle.

Negative mindsets need not apply for prolonged fasting. I cannot stress this enough. We should approach prolonged fasting with a rather open mindset. This is because it involves throwing conventional wisdom out of the window, but also because we do not know everything there is to know about it just yet.

So what *do* we know about it?

SURVIVAL, BURNING FAT, AND SAVING MUSCLE

Each of us needs what nature gives us,

when nature gives it.

- MARCUS AURELIUS

The ability to eat whenever we like represents but an evolutionary *millisecond*. For most of our story on this earth, we had to hunt and gather our own food, so periods of food scarcity were common. Mother Nature has designed us with survival in mind. As a human being, you possess several survival mechanisms. And when you fast, you call them into action.

The common perception is that if you are to fast for longer than a day, it will drain you of all your muscles and physical capabilities. But this could not be further from the truth. If evolution had not genetically programmed us to perform at a high level while fasting, then humanity would not have survived for very long. It's that simple. And I'll prove it.

Conventional wisdom suggests that fasting is a terrible idea and will make us weak and lethargic. However, this notion only makes sense if we limit ourselves to the false belief system that states we must eat frequently to survive. As we have seen in the last chapter, eating frequently for energy is nonsense. To really understand how we adapt to prolonged fasting, we must approach it with a fresh perspective.

It's time for a paradigm shift.

Fasting increases the production of growth hormone (GH). According to a study from the University of Virginia Medical School, two days of fasting can trigger as much as a *fivefold* increase. In another study, Peter Kerndt and his team from the University of California monitored a man who embarked on a forty-day fast. They found that GH production kept increasing until the twenty-sixth day of the fast. At this stage, it was producing at *thirteen* times the normal rate. GH therapy, which involves injections of the hormone, has anti-aging properties. But it comes with some undesirable side effects, such as an increased risk of heart problems. Why not try fasting therapy instead? It boosts GH and offers all the benefits with none of the side effects. It will be a lot cheaper too. And it doesn't involve any needles. Emulating authentic patterns of human behaviour is the way forward. Mother Nature knows what's up.

I know what you're thinking.

Fasting will turn me into the Hulk!

But it is not the case. The reality is not so sexy. But it *is* fascinating. First, a few words on growth hormone.

Fasting stimulates GH, but it will not create new muscle tissue. Building muscle requires training and energy from food. During fasting, GH serves as Mother Nature's defence mechanism, as it prevents the breakdown of muscle mass and stimulates burning fat for fuel.

Think of it this way. Imagine our friend Zug has gone a whole day without food. He is facing a period of food scarcity, and dinner looks like it will be hard to find. To end the food scarcity, he will need energy, which comes from burning fat, and he will also need his precious muscle and strength to hunt and gather. If we were to burn muscle instead of fat during periods of fasting, then we would not have been able to survive for as long we have. Mother Nature knows the deal.

Many people are adamant that fasting will burn muscle, but in reality, the opposite occurs. Fasting directly *prevents* the burning of muscle and *prioritizes* the burning of fat for fuel instead. If we did not have such a response in our locker, then fasting would be tricky. In a study from the Aarhus University Hospital in Denmark, researchers showed that a *lack* of growth hormone during prolonged fasting could increase muscle breakdown by around 50%. During prolonged fasting, GH saves muscle mass, and in doing so, it saves lives. This surge in production is a necessary adaptation to ensure that we can continue to function optimally and rise to the challenge of combatting a period of food scarcity. Without this adaptation, we lose the battle of survival. And the story of humanity would have ended with our mate Zug. GH keeps us strong and ready during a fast. It may also keep us looking *young*.

We mentioned the anti-aging potential of GH earlier, and if we consult the data, we see this both in a physical and a mental sense. GH improves several markers of happiness and psychological capabilities, and clinicians have used it to treat various mood and memory disorders. Happiness keeps you looking young, as they say. Research has also shown GH to benefit mental awareness and motivation, both are qualities that would have been useful in navigating a period of food scarcity. On an aesthetic level, GH maintains healthy skin, nails and hair. And nothing says anti-aging more than a natural glow. Maintaining muscle mass, a key function of GH, will also help to slow down the aging process. Keeping your body strong and mobile makes getting older a breeze. GH plays a key role in living healthier for longer, which explains why scientists regard it as the hormone of longevity. But like I said before, GH therapy comes with side effects.

And it's not cheap. However, with fasting therapy, there are no side effects. Just a thicker wallet. How beautiful it is, that during a time of perceived danger (food scarcity in this case) the body produces more of the very hormone responsible for living longer. When the chips are down, Mother Nature has our back.

Prolonged fasting does not burn muscle. When you realise that you need not eat frequently for energy, it opens up a whole new avenue of understanding. Mother Nature has blessed us with various survival mechanisms that allow us to navigate periods of food scarcity, and we can activate them by fasting. Today, we are lucky enough not to have to worry about survival, so we can use these mechanisms to benefit other areas of life instead.

In this context, we can use fasting to slow down the aging process, prevent muscle breakdown, and keep us looking fresh.

FEELING FULL, METABOLIC MOOD SWINGS, AND ROCKET FUEL

Whenever you find yourself on the side of the majority,
it is time to pause and reflect.

- MARK TWAIN

Three common misconceptions of prolonged fasting:

I'll be too hungry.

It will damage my metabolism.

And I won't have any energy.

None of these are true. Not even *remotely*.

Let me explain.

In the second part, we discussed the role that ghrelin plays in hunger. Within this discussion, we looked at a study that measured ghrelin during a twenty-four-hour fast. And we saw that it comes in waves. Hunger arrives, sticks around for half an hour, and then disappears. Prolonged fasting follows a similar pattern, but there is an important difference. Researchers from Aarhus University Hospital in Denmark monitored levels of ghrelin during an *eighty-four hour* fast. As expected, hunger came in waves. But these waves became *less* pronounced as the fast went on. For example, the researchers observed the highest spike of ghrelin on day one of the fast. And the average level of Ghrelin decreased with each day of fasting. Contrary to what many people may have thought would happen, hunger was becoming *less* of an issue the longer the fast went on. The average ghrelin reading at the *end* of the fast was much lower than at the *start* of the fast, suggesting that a long fast will *reduce* appetite, rather than stimulate it. Hunger is not an issue during prolonged fasting. In fact, the longer that a person fasts, the less hunger they feel. This can be a strange concept to grasp, as it seems counterintuitive. If I'm not eating, *surely* I will feel hungrier? But the reality is quite the opposite. During prolonged fasting, hunger almost *disappears*.

To have full control over hunger makes prolonged fasting enjoyable, but also empowering. Detaching yourself from the grip of hunger makes you realise just how much time and energy you spend on food. Not only eating it, but thinking about it too. In this sense, fasting is freedom. And it opens many doors that we once had locked. That's hunger sorted, so let's move on to the metabolism.

Many people believe that fasting will damage or slow down the metabolism. But again, this is not true. When people think of the metabolism slowing down, what they mean is the metabolic rate decreases, or the amount of energy we spend goes down. A popular belief is that fasting will put us into some kind of *starvation mode*, in which we decrease our metabolic rate so much that we stop losing fat. This is nonsense. And you will see why. Let's look at what the research can tell us about changes to our metabolic rate during prolonged fasting.

Before we begin, remember that everything we do has a *price* in terms of energy. We don't just spend energy on moving around, but also on things like our digestive system and our level of concentration.

During the first few days of prolonged fasting, our metabolic rate increases. We spend more energy until around seventy hours of fasting. At which point, our rate of energy expenditure levels out. It often surprises people to find out that fasting for longer than a day can *increase* metabolic rate. But it's super simple when we frame it in the evolutionary context. During the first few days of fasting, the body shifts into a *higher gear*, increasing energy levels and activating various survival mechanisms. To do this, the body needs to spend more energy. Think of energy as a currency. When we fast, the body spends more to guarantee survival. And so our metabolic rate increases to compensate.

But the metabolic rate cannot stay elevated; otherwise, we would burn through our stored fuel reserves far too quickly. The metabolic rate increases only until around three days of fasting, at which point it begins to go in the other direction. If we frame this trend in the evolutionary context, it seems logical. If three days have passed and there is still no food in sight, it would be unwise for the body to continue functioning in this higher gear, because it is more costly in terms of energy and will burn through all of the fuel reserve. After three days of fasting, Mother Nature realises that we may face a far lengthier spell of food scarcity than imagined. So it instructs the body to dial back on its energy spending to ensure survival for the longest duration of time. The decrease in the metabolic rate after three days of fasting reflects the adaptive mechanisms taking place as the body prepares for a potentially very long time without food.

We also have to consider the fact that after three days without eating, we will use fewer bodily functions. So the price to keep the lights on is much lower. For example, after three days of fasting, our digestive system, which has quite a substantial energy price tag, is more or less dormant. We need not spend as much energy after three days of fasting, and we reflect this in the changes to our metabolic rate.

You might wonder *why* our metabolic rate increases so much during the first few days of a fast. This has to do with our energy levels, and it provides a convenient path to another popular misconception of fasting.

Many claim that fasting will deteriorate energy levels to where a person cannot function anymore. But this is not a science-based view. And the reality is quite the opposite. Although there will be a point at which physical and mental vigour can decline during a fast, it arrives much later than most think. Prolonged fasting may well make you feel more energetic than ever. And perhaps even *euphoric*.

Remember, we need not eat frequently for energy. The body is still generating and consuming energy to function and survive during periods of fasting. This energy just comes in the form of stored body fat. The body has already packed several lunches to prepare for this journey, and it is more than happy to use them. In part two, we discussed how shorter periods of fasting can make us feel more alert, but during prolonged fasting, energy levels can *skyrocket*.

The important factor here is the difference between our conscious understanding of the situation we find ourselves in and how our body and brain will interpret it. Evolution has programmed our genes blindly, but they always win. For example, let's say that you have been fasting for twenty-four hours. You know that you can break your fast whenever you feel like it. There is plenty of food available, and it's easy to get. You are very much fasting out of choice, rather than out of necessity because of food scarcity. Or out of fear from a scary looking sabre-toothed tiger prowling the savannah. However, the crucial difference is that your brain is none the wiser. For all the brain knows, you are in a dark cave during monsoon season. Lost in the Amazon with a wooden spear and no food in sight. Or sitting on a Barcelona balcony with a plethora of tapas options downstairs. The brain responds to *food scarcity*, as this is how it perceives the situation of fasting. The brain does not know that you could have a feast delivered to your door within twenty minutes. And this is the reason we experience such hormonal adaptations that help us survive.

As we increase the length of a fast, the brain interprets this situation as a period of food scarcity becoming longer and a threat to our survival. Therefore, Mother Nature ramps up her response, and she expresses this through an increased rate of fat burning. This supplies us with more energy, which we can use in our quest to *end* the food scarcity. Another survival response to the situation, and something that sends energy levels through the roof, is the release of *catecholamines*. (pronounced cat - e - chol - amine)

Though they may sound like a Latin American punk band, the catecholamines are responsible for stimulating the release of adrenaline, dopamine and norepinephrine. When the body releases the catecholamines, we feel *alive*. And this is Mother Nature's way of preparing us for survival.

The catecholamine that we will focus on in this section is norepinephrine (nuh-reh-puh-neh-fruhn). Think of it as Mother Nature's *rocket fuel*.

Norepinephrine makes us feel alive. It heightens alertness, makes us super perceptive of the environment, and gives us laser-like focus. If you have ever embarked on a prolonged fast and felt sharper than usual, norepinephrine played a part. It also plays an important role in the consolidation and retrieval of memories. Research shows that norepinephrine is key in the ability to respond to sudden changes in the environment. During periods of food scarcity, Zug would have had to have been alert and able to read the environment with precision. He would have had to react to sudden changes and shift into a higher gear. We are the descendants of those who could react to subtle and sudden changes in their surroundings during periods of food scarcity. Therefore, it only makes sense that these adaptations occur during prolonged fasting. Stimulating norepinephrine helps us to shift into a *higher gear* and supercharges our levels of perception and alertness.

Researchers from the University of Vienna found that norepinephrine production skyrocketed after twenty-fours of fasting. And levels continued to increase all the way through an eighty-hour fast. The rise in norepinephrine follows a very similar pattern to the increase of the metabolic rate we discussed earlier. Coincidence? I think not. Considering that norepinephrine makes us more energetic, the connection between norepinephrine and metabolic rate makes sense. If we feel more energetic, we are spending more energy. And our metabolic rate will increase. When we stimulate norepinephrine, the brain shifts the body into a higher gear. And the metabolic rate increases. Something else that is interesting is the research suggesting that high levels of norepinephrine can make you feel *euphoric*.

It was a rare sunny afternoon in Greater London and I had made the most of it by taking the dogs out for a swift stroll. I stopped at a bridge, and looked up to the sky, which had adopted that pink hue typical of the transition between day and night. A wave came over me. Not of hunger, but of tranquility. I felt a laser-like focus on the present moment. Rather than just bumble along listening to music or thinking about some hypothetical scenario, I was now scanning the landscape with great interest. I could notice things I had never cared for, like the different trees, the perfect sky, or how my dogs interacted with each other and their environment. Even the range of scents on offer became interesting. In this moment, there was no anxiety, guilt, regret or worry anywhere in my psyche. Only wonder and joy. This is what I refer to as *borderline euphoria*.

But what made this walk different? On this occasion, I was *deep* into the fasted state. About seventy-two hours. And according to the data, norepinephrine is rather high at seventy-two hours. Who knew that survival could feel so incredible?

Another activity that stimulates norepinephrine is exercise.

Maybe you have felt that sensation of feeling alert and alive following intense exercise. Perhaps you have even felt euphoric too. The brain could interpret intense exercise as a potential threat to survival. For all it knows, instead of doing laps on the treadmill or scoring a screamer in the last minute of the game, you could be running away from a sabre-toothed tiger.

Many think it is inconceivable that prolonged fasting could increase energy levels. But when we frame it in an evolutionary context, it seems logical. With our friend Zug, who lived before supermarkets and fridges, finding food was a task that required a great deal of energy and concentration. If his energy levels were to deteriorate without food, then finding it would be difficult. To find food, he *needed* a boost. Otherwise, he would perish. We are the descendants of the humans that survived. And the ones that survived were those who could shift into a *higher gear* during periods of food scarcity and fasting.

Fasting is Mother Nature's most potent stimulant. Nothing gets you going like a little food scarcity. *Up and at 'em!*

It is also worth considering what is happening to us on a surface level. Food consumes a lot of mental energy. It's not just the act of sitting down to eat, but all the planning, purchasing, cooking and cleaning that comes along with it. Not having to think about food liberates a substantial amount of mental energy that we can invest in other areas of life. During prolonged fasting, we have no choice but to focus on other things aside from food. And this can be a transformative experience. Therapeutic, even.

Prolonged fasting.

Energy is sky high.

Hunger is under control.

And the metabolism is secure.

You may even feel *euphoric* too.

KETONES, RADICAL COWBOYS, AND DAVE'S FENCE

Abstinence and fasting cure many a complaint.

- DANISH PROVERB

To use stored fat as fuel, the body must break it down and convert it into ketone bodies*, which are a source of energy. After around four hours from our last meal, ketone production increases at a steady rate until around twenty-four hours of fasting. At which point, the rate of production skyrockets. This continues until around seventy-two hours of fasting. By this stage, the body is running primarily on ketones, also known as being in a state of *ketosis*, and the rate of production levels out.

When there is no glucose from food available, the body can use ketones as fuel. They can also cross the blood-brain barrier to power the most energy-demanding organ that we have: the brain. This is how humans have been able to survive long periods of food scarcity. If we could not use our stored fat as fuel to power our brain, then we would have perished a long time ago. Research has also shown that ketone bodies inhibit the breakdown of muscle mass, which would have been a key component of our survival during periods of food scarcity. For many years, scientists have regarded ketone bodies as a

---

*Ketone bodies are produced by the liver from fatty acids and used as an energy source when glucose is not readily available.

mere back-up energy source that we use only in emergency situations, such as starvation. However, emerging research suggests that they can be a superior fuel source for the brain. Compared to glucose, ketone bodies supply more energy per unit of oxygen consumed, and they do so at a faster rate. They may be a *cleaner* source of energy, too.

Various animal studies have shown that metabolizing ketone bodies for fuel can produce less free radicals, which will have important implications for our overall health and longevity. You may wonder what on earth a *free radical* is. Let me tell you. It's a *cowboy*. And to explain what I mean by that, I will have to go back to basics and ask: *what are we made of?*

Obviously, there's skin, bones, muscles and blood and whatnot. But what makes these things? The simple answer is *cells*. Trillions of cells make up the human body. Skin cells, bone cells, muscle cells, blood cells, nerve cells and plenty more. Molecules are the building blocks of the cell, and this is where the story of the free radical begins. Molecules are works of art that comprise pairs of electrons. When the molecule has the correct number of electron pairs that it requires, it can perform its duty within the biological community. However, if just one of those electrons goes missing, then the molecule becomes unstable. Losing an electron causes the molecule to feel disillusioned and lose its way. It rejects conventional life and follows the path of the free radical.

Not all cowboys are born cowboys. Sometimes it can take an unfortunate event, like losing an electron that they once held dear, to cause them to lose faith and choose the path of radical cowboyism. Free radicals are unstable, highly reactive, and do not follow any rules. In true cowboy fashion, the free radicals will hold up other molecules at gunpoint and demand that they give up their electrons. When a free radical forces another molecule to surrender its electrons, this molecule becomes imbalanced and disheartened, which leads them into becoming a free radical. If this cycle continues for too long, it will cause irreversible damage to our DNA. So, it's clear we want little to do with the free radicals. But ironically, they are constantly being formed in the body, as we need a certain amount of them to survive. The cowboys also protect the town from invasion, as we can use the free radicals to kill bacteria trying to infect us. The free radicals will always be around in some quantity; we just need to manage them in the correct way. A few cowboys can maintain order in the town and keep everything ticking over. But too many will cause havoc.

If you have ever wondered why we need antioxidants, it's because of the free radicals. The antioxidants are the good guys, as they donate electrons to the wayward free radicals, which neutralises them. They are the selfless heroes that talk sense into the cowboys and put them back on the straight and narrow. It's all about establishing a balance. When the cowboys outnumber the antioxidants, the result is *oxidative stress*. Too much of this stress can lead to arthritis, heart disease, infertility and various neurodegenerative disorders such as Parkinson's and Alzheimer's. Therefore, keeping oxidative stress at bay will be key in optimising health and longevity. Consuming more antioxidants through diet is an option, but antioxidants in the form of supplements can be harmful if we take them in excessive doses. Remember, it's all about the *balance*. If the free radicals outnumber the antioxidants, there will be serious problems. But there can also be complications if the antioxidants outnumber the free radicals. So the most effective strategy will be to reduce the number of free radicals the body produces in the first place, thus reducing the need for more antioxidants. Fasting allows the body plenty of time to use the cleaner fuel source of ketone bodies, reducing free radicals and protecting us from oxidative stress.

Many people report that being in a state of ketosis and running on ketone bodies gives them an *edge*. They feel sharp with mental clarity and laser-like focus and are more productive and positive overall. I recall a meme on social media of a bear surfing a huge wave with a shark as a surfboard, screaming and firing a machine gun. The caption? *'This is what it feels like to be in ketosis'.*

Say no more. Can't argue with a meme, after all.

Remember Dave from football? According to Dave, the only thing that got him off of his backside to paint his fence was being in a state of ketosis. Many people claim that being in ketosis is like having superpowers, but clinical research is still in its infancy. Accera is a biotechnology company that develops therapeutic drugs for neurodegenerative diseases. Ketone bodies have shown promise in the realm of brain health, so researchers from Accera experimented with them. Their study was published in the journal *Neurobiology of Aging*, and they found that ketones increased the level of memory recall in adults with memory disorders. We know that ketones make positive movements in the brain, but we do not know to what extent. Mystery still clouds the subject, but there are promising indications. It may sound odd, but many people, including myself, will use fasting as a tool to negotiate busy periods that require high levels of concentration. If I need to be sharp for a certain task, I always make sure I'm deep into the fasted state and running on ketones.

Ketones are a clean fuel source that may carry several health benefits and boost productivity. They could be the next big thing. So get them while you can. The best part about them? They are easy to get. You don't have to pay through the nose, subscribe to any program or, God forbid, do anything illegal.

All you have to do is stop eating for a while.

CLEANING UP YOUR ROOM, YEAST, AND AUTOPHAGY

Keep only those things that speak to your heart.

Then take the plunge and discard all the rest.

By doing this, you can reset your life and embark on a new lifestyle.

- MARIE KONDŌ

オートファジー

We construct the word *autophagy* from the Latin words *auto*, meaning self, and *phagous*, which means eating. Yes, you read that correctly. Autophagy means *self-eating*.

This sounds undesirable, but in reality, it is a powerful healing process. Don't forget, cells make up our entire body, and this process of self-eating refers to the consumption of any harmful or obsolete cells. Eating these cells provides energy which the body can use to generate new cells or repair existing ones. Forget the cucumbers and face cream, the best detox comes from within.

Everything in the body, including the digestive system, uses energy. When we allow the digestive system a break during periods of fasting, it liberates energetic resources that the body can invest in other areas. We can use these resources to enhance our internal regulation by regenerating cells and fighting disease. The primary aim of autophagy is to clean our cells and recycle anything that we do not need. As I'm sure we all know, cleaning is a task that we should *never* ignore. The wonderful and slightly mesmerising Japanese organising consultant Marie Kondo, said it best:

The objective of cleaning is not just to clean, but to feel happiness living within that environment.

They may not know it, but autophagy and Marie Kondo share a similar aim. Autophagy does not just aim to clean, but to fight disease and keep us healthy too. Factors that will make us feel happy while living within our physiological environment.

Autophagy is like an upgrade from the app store; it eliminates the bugs and improves the features. Much like an upgrade, autophagy requires a *restart*. If there are too many programs open, it is hard to download an upgrade. Likewise, if the digestion of food is occupying our body, it will struggle to focus on autophagy. Upgrades require energy, focus and peace, and autophagy requires periods of fasting. Let's consider the evolutionary framework. Fasting activates several physiological adaptations that make survival the top priority. The function of autophagy is to remove life-threatening faulty cells from our body and protect us from various diseases and disorders. Therefore, it promotes longevity and reduces the number of risks posed to our health, thus increasing our likelihood of survival. When survival is the primary concern, the body will not destroy the very mechanisms that promote long-term health. That makes little sense. Instead, it will *amplify* these mechanisms. Autophagy responds to certain hormetic stressors, such as calorie restriction and exercise, but fasting may bring autophagy to a whole new level.

You can answer the most basic and important questions about the nature of life through yeasts.

- YOSHINORI OHSUMI

In 2016, the Nobel Foundation awarded Japanese cell biologist Yoshinori Ohsumi the Nobel Prize in Physiology or Medicine for his studies on yeast that led to breakthrough discoveries on autophagy. Ohsumi's work explained the mechanisms behind Autophagy and provided a powerful molecular tool kit that scientists all over the world can use to study this phenomenon. Amidst all the promise of autophagy, it is easy to forget that research is still in its infancy. Scientists find it incredibly complicated to measure autophagy in humans, and as a result clinical research is sparse. The findings from lab animals, however, are crystal clear: rodents who fast experience *profound* autophagy. Studies show that mice subjected to prolonged fasting can regenerate their entire immune system and greatly reduce cancer risk. Human studies, however, are lacking. We *know* fasting stimulates autophagy, but how long we should fast for or exactly what to expect are matters that remain somewhat mysterious. However, if we consider some other elements of fasting, we can shed light on the matter.

Prolonged fasting increases growth hormone production, which, as we know, serves various functions during a fast. In autophagy, there is one that is crucial: the key role that GH plays in cellular repair. One study from the University of Texas Southwestern Medical Center found that elevating levels of GH in mice stimulated the process of autophagy. Further research from the University of Chicago showed that GH activated a gene critical for the body's tissues to heal and regenerate. While the surge of GH serves primarily as a defence mechanism preventing muscle breakdown, it also provides autophagy with the tools to repair existing cells and generate new ones. Consider that GH production surges during prolonged fasting, and we can assume that stimulating profound autophagy in humans would require a few days of fasting. Regardless of how long it takes to get it going, autophagy could be a *game-changer* for humanity. Although it may seem like a simple process, autophagy is complex and there are several layers to it, so it will take some time to unpack. The future is bright. But we are not there yet.

Many people will fast for a specific time to stimulate autophagy, but remember it is unclear how long or how often we should fast to optimise the process. Don't hold yourself hostage to a certain time frame in the name of autophagy. Rather, work the fast around your lifestyle and how you feel.

The subject of autophagy has attracted a lot of interest in recent years, and as a result many have seen a business opportunity. Remember, it's still early days in terms of research, so be sceptical of anyone trying to sell products on the claim that they enhance autophagy. There is a lot we don't know, but we *do* know that calorie restriction, exercise, and fasting all benefit autophagy, so don't worry about anything else. For now.

Stay open-minded, but always remember to dig deeper and look for the evidence.

Prolonged fasting is like the therapeutic use of certain psychedelic compounds. We know there is a benefit, but we are unclear on the optimal dose or frequency. Fasting triggers autophagy in humans which *could* be a game changer of epic proportions, but let's not get carried away just yet.

Autophagy is Mother Nature's ways of taking us to the app store to give us an upgrade and get rid of any bugs. The potential is immense, but we are still learning.

Aa, sugoi kirei jan!

WHAT TO EXPECT

The very act of eating can be exhausting;
it takes a lot of energy to digest food.
When the body is freed from that chore,
it naturally feels lighter and much more vibrant.

- ALLAN COTT

Prolonged fasting can be a mixed bag. Every experience has the potential to be different. But here are some common themes you can expect.

The first thing you will notice is the *freedom*. The realisation of just how much time and energy food takes up from your daily life will come crashing to the surface. Liberated from food, you now have total freedom. For a few days at least. With all this time and mental energy, you will get a lot done. And you may even experience periods of deep reflection. A time for introspection. Both in a physiological sense, with the body burning fat and ramping up autophagy, and from a mental perspective.

Bedtime can be tricky. You will find getting to sleep is difficult, and you will sleep a lot less. Despite this, the symptoms of a poor night's sleep do not appear. You will wake up feeling well-rested and ready to go. Energy levels will be high, you will feel alert, and productivity will be through the roof. During prolonged fasting, the mind is razor sharp. Many people experience a deeper level of perception about their environment. You will notice things you have never seen before. Perhaps on the way to work, about a colleague, or even in yourself. Fasting allows you to step out of the box and observe life differently. There will be lots of positive emotions. During prolonged fasting, you will feel happy. Perhaps even euphoric.

Prolonged fasting sheds away anything that you do not need and tunes you into the best and most efficient version of yourself. The reason it does this is simple. The best version of yourself has the best chance of surviving a period of food scarcity. Everything comes back to *survival*, which is why you feel so alert, productive, and positive. There is no time for laziness, self-doubt or procrastination when survival is on the line. And perhaps that is the most important thing that we must remember: it's a survival adaptation. So it's also a stressor to the system. While it can be an exhilarating experience, it is not something I would do too often. When we fast for a long period, we are asking a lot from the body. Don't overdo it.

Prolonged fasting is not without its risks. There are some things we must remember and take care of, which we shall discuss in the next section. But I warn you, it might get *salty*.

ROMANS, ELECTROLYTES, AND TAKING YOUR TIME

You are an explorer,

and you represent our species,

and the greatest good you can do is to bring back a new idea,

because our world is endangered by the absence of good ideas.

Our world is in crisis because of the absence of consciousness.

- TERENCE MCKENNA

Let's talk about *salt*.

Do you know the origin of the word *salary*?

Once upon a time, salt was worth its weight in gold. The Roman empire often paid its soldiers in salt (known then as *sal*), and this led to the word *salary*.

You would not be best pleased if I presented you with a bag of salt after a working week, but the Romans were not mad, because we need salt to stay alive.

Our very distant ancestors lived in the sea, and as a result, their bodies became adapted to a salty environment. Humans have lived on land for millions of years, but we still need salt to live, as it is crucial for maintaining an adequate blood volume and pressure. Have you ever wondered why the taste of salt is pleasurable? Perhaps it's an evolutionary adaptation to ensure that we seek it out and consume enough to survive. The mainstream media have demonised salt, and although too much can be harmful, too *little* is perhaps more dangerous. Sodium is the primary component of salt, and this is an essential nutrient that keeps our heart pumping blood and replenishes the physiological balance of the body. If we do not consume enough sodium, it can cause the life-threatening condition of hyponatremia. The reason I'm discussing salt with such passion is because of the key role it plays in regulating our electrolyte balance. When we fast for prolonged periods, we lose electrolytes. You may have heard of electrolytes before, perhaps through the various marketing campaigns of several sugar-laden sports drinks, but have you ever wondered *what* they are?

Electrolytes are necessary for several essential processes in the body, including muscle contraction, nerve impulses, and regular heart rate.

The four major electrolytes we will focus on are **sodium**, **chloride**, **potassium** and **magnesium**.

The body expresses an electrolyte imbalance through headaches or fatigue. However, there are various other symptoms, such as muscle cramps, extreme thirst, and in the more extreme cases: elevated heart rate and heart palpitations. During intense exercise when we lose large quantities of water through sweat, electrolytes can become imbalanced. An example of this is when you see footballers cramping up during periods of extra time, as cramping is a signal to communicate that electrolytes are running low. However, electrolytes can also become imbalanced during prolonged fasting. When we fast, we are flushing out a substantial amount of fluid, and with that loss of fluid, we lose electrolytes. Ample hydration during a fast is essential, but the electrolyte balance is also important. During the shorter fasting periods involved in an intermittent fasting schedule, one need not worry too much about the electrolyte balance. However, it is something that we must manage during a prolonged fast that is longer than twenty-four hours in duration. In most cases, a pinch of Himalayan pink salt will do the trick. You can either mix it with water (it dissolves best in sparkling water, but be careful as it can bubble), or you can place a few crystals under your tongue. Many reject eating salt, but during a fast, it is a welcome taste. Himalayan pink salt is a good source of sodium and chloride, which are the electrolytes we lose the quickest during fasting and exercise. If we fast for a day or two, then pink salt alone will be sufficient. However, if we are to fast for longer, or feel symptoms of electrolyte depletion, then we must consider where we are at regarding potassium and magnesium. Pink salt contains potassium and magnesium, but only in trace amounts. It is straightforward to keep these two electrolytes replenished, as there are plenty of inexpensive supplements that offer the full range of electrolytes (just make sure they don't contain sugar.) Regulating electrolyte balance and staying well hydrated are *essential* for anyone looking to fast for a prolonged period.

I once received a message containing a photo of an electrolyte powder sachet with the sender asking, 'is this okay during a fast?'

Upon closer inspection of the ingredients, although the electrolytes *were* present, there was also 13.5 grams of dextrose, which is another way of saying *sugar*.

I suspect that they designed it with the endurance athlete in mind, perhaps a long-distance runner or cyclist, who is relying on glucose for fuel rather than fat. Said athlete can convert dextrose to fuel in the form of glucose, but we are interested in using *stored fat* for energy, not glucose.

For the high sugar content, an electrolyte powder like this *will* break the fast and is not a good idea.

I assume it was expensive too.

Always read the label.

During prolonged periods of fasting, avoid intense training. Working out is not off limits; we just need to be careful. If you have to go, keep it light. We must remind ourselves of two important factors. The first is that during a prolonged fast, the body will not be growing new muscle tissue, so there is no point in lifting heavy. Second, we are already burning fat and creating a sizeable calorie deficit by fasting for so long, so we need not worry about doing cardio to burn more calories.

Take it easy.

If you want to stay active during a fast, then get walking.

We also need to address the matter of consuming calories during a prolonged fast. It sounds silly to discuss, but some people feel inclined to consume something small to enjoy a little flavour or as a crutch to keep them going. However, when embarking on a prolonged fast, it is very important not to *cheat* by eating or drinking even a tiny amount of calories. Allow me to clarify why that is.

Has eating or drinking a small amount of calories ever satisfied anyone? The opposite is true for most people. Consuming a small amount of calories will *open* the floodgates of hunger, rather than secure them. Fasting is easier when we do it without crutches. Remember that everything in the body has a price in terms of energy, and the digestive system is rather expensive to maintain. When we eat something, we call our digestive organs to action, and they all require fuel to take part. Consider it as the price of doing business with your digestive system. However, when we fast for prolonged periods of time, the digestive system goes into something of a dormant state, because we do not need it if we are not eating. Let us not underestimate Mother Nature. During periods of food scarcity, the brain recognises there is no need to keep the lights on in the digestive system, so it dials down the energy demand. We need to preserve energy for as long as possible during periods of food scarcity, so spending energy to keep the digestive system functioning would not be a wise investment. Under the astute financial guidance of Mother Nature, the brain is far too clever to commit such a schoolboy error and spend energy on something that is unnecessary. This would also help to explain why our metabolic rate decreases after three complete days of fasting. The cost of keeping the lights on is a lot less.

Imagine you go on a month-long holiday to the Canary Islands. Would you leave the lights on in your house? No. You would turn everything off and avoid wasting energy in your home while you're not there. If we eat while our digestive system is in this dormant state, we are waking it up and kicking it into gear again, and this costs energy. The problem is, we are turning the whole system on again just to process a tiny amount of calories, which makes no sense. Like driving your car to get petrol at a station that is 100 miles away with only 60 miles worth of petrol left in the tank. The body now has a higher energy demand to power the digestive system, but there is no energy coming in, so it will have to pay for it by taking from other processes, which can lower energy levels, increase hunger and make the fast uncomfortable. It's not worth it. If you want to eat, eat and enjoy it. Likewise, if you want to fast, then fast and enjoy it. We do not permit fence-sitting in the realm of prolonged fasting.

Let's move on to discuss *breaking* the prolonged fast. As Mahatma Gandhi said, 'more caution and perhaps more restraint are necessary in breaking a fast than in keeping it.'

Breaking the fast is important, and a failure to do so has negative consequences. We must take care when reintroducing food to a dormant digestive system. Would you rather soothing birdsong wakes you up, or your father-in-law breaks your slumber by launching a bucket of cold water in your general direction? If the body has been fasting for several days, we must wake up the digestive system throughout gradual stages. The longer we fast, the longer we will need to spend breaking the fast. Start off with transition foods: foods easy to digest without refined sugar. Bone broth, soups, celery juice and items of that ilk are ideal. As we gradually work our way up to eating large meals again, we must take care to reintroduce foods. In very extreme cases, the rapid reintroduction of food following a prolonged period of fasting and failure to manage the electrolyte balance leads to fatal consequences.

Scientists observed refeeding syndrome at the end of the Second World War when Japanese prisoners of war experienced adverse effects with the rapid reintroduction of solid foods following the starvation they had endured. Rapidly reintroducing food is problematic, but an electrolyte deficiency also has consequences. Without electrolytes the body cannot deal with the food being reintroduced. When we fast for prolonged periods of time, the body enters a state of deep ketosis, in which it adapts to metabolising fat for fuel. If we suddenly shift from this metabolic state by introducing carbohydrate-based foods, it causes the body to release a flood of insulin to handle the digestion. This metabolic process requires a substantial amount of electrolytes, and if we are deficient in them, there *will* be consequences. We reserve this classification for somewhat extreme circumstances, but it still serves to underline the importance of electrolytes and the reintroduction of food following prolonged fasting.

Keep the electrolytes balanced and take care with the reintroduction of food. We cannot underestimate how important these elements are.

Just like a car, we cannot take off in fifth gear; instead, we must start in first and ascend through the gears with composure.

TOO EASY: A WORD OF CAUTION

Prolonged fasting is easier than most imagine, and it comes with a special energy. Hunger dissipates, energy levels stabilise and the mind sharpens, complemented with an underlying sensation that I can only describe as borderline euphoria. This sounds positive, but for some, it can lead to negative developments. For example, those with an eating disorder or an unhealthy relationship with their body image. Prolonged fasting can turn into another form of abuse by punishment for eating too much or doing something wrong. These people can become *obsessed* with losing weight, and the ease of fasting allows them to take it to extreme measures. In such cases, prolonged fasting is a slippery slope. If a person is underweight, has an unhealthy relationship with their body image, or a history of disordered eating, then they *must* avoid prolonged fasting. No exceptions.

The benefits will *not* outweigh the detrimental impact it will have on such a person.

HUNGRY LIONS DON'T SLEEP

Sleep can be an issue during prolonged fasting. However, although many people find they sleep *less*, they do not report the usual symptoms of a poor night's sleep. In fact, they find that during prolonged periods of fasting, they sleep for much less than usual but they wake up full of energy and raring to go. This is peculiar, but when we frame it an evolutionary context, it becomes clear.

During periods of food scarcity, several survival mechanisms activate and the body adapts to the situation. Minimising sleep and maximising wakefulness is one of those mechanisms. If Zug was busy sleeping, then he is not finding food. If we look in nature, the only time that animals voluntarily deprive themselves of sleep is during periods of food scarcity. Prolonged fasting stimulates norepinephrine, which increases alertness and energy levels, but *orexin* also plays a key role in the shortening of sleep, as it regulates wakefulness. Prolonged fasting raises orexin, contributing to that strange sensation of waking up feeling fresh despite having slept less than usual. During prolonged fasting, Mother Nature allows us to operate at full capacity with less sleep, so we spend more time awake finding food.

Although it may feel like we can function optimally with less sleep during prolonged fasting, it is a *temporary* adaptation. The ill-effects of sleep deprivation still apply if we sleep less during prolonged fasting, so it is important not to get carried away with this energetic sensation. Even if it *feels* like we can go without, we must still treat sleep as a top priority. Regarding getting to sleep, some methods that have helped me are sauna sessions, baths with Epsom salts, being as active as possible during the day and plenty of reading before bedtime. During prolonged fasting, it feels like we need not sleep as much, but remember it is a temporary survival mechanism.

Sleep must *always* be a priority.

If you begin to feel bad during a prolonged fast for whatever reason, just eat. It's all about enjoying the process. If at any point it becomes unpleasant, then reassess the situation, and do not feel as if you have to complete the fast duration that you had planned on.

It's just a number.

How you feel will *always* be paramount.

SUMMARY

Fasting today makes the food good tomorrow.

- GERMAN PROVERB

Not only are we well equipped to survive during periods of prolonged fasting but to *thrive* too.

Mother Nature has blessed us with the mechanisms to cope with and navigate prolonged periods of food scarcity. The question is, where does prolonged fasting fit into a healthy lifestyle? Answers to this question will vary depending on who you ask, but there are a few things we should consider. First, as we have already discussed, we still don't know enough to prescribe fasting with the goal of optimising autophagy. Perhaps three days of fasting once every quarter of the year are plenty, or maybe one whole day of fasting per month will do the trick. It is still unclear what the optimal approach is, so why worry about optimal? Let's just focus on what works for *us*.

For those with a lot of weight to lose, prolonged fasting presents itself as a useful tool. It makes sense that if one has plenty of stored energy then fasting for a prolonged period of time would put it to good use. But a balanced approach will always be optimal. Working on making small lifestyle modifications and establishing a healthy balance between fasting and feeding will always be a more sustainable method. Promoting prolonged fasting for fat loss alone is unwise. And in the wrong hands, it is a dangerous tool, like someone who is attempting to mask an eating disorder for example. Fat loss comes from our long-term habits and our lifestyle. Relying on prolonged fasting to make progress in terms of fat loss is *not* the way.

Let's approach prolonged fasting with an open mind. I believe that prolonged fasting unlocks something profound from within the human psyche, and in a world teeming with materialistic distractions, this is precious. Fasting allows us to connect with the experience of being alive on a much deeper level.

And if you care to join me for the next part, you will see why.

Part Five

FASTING AND THE BRAIN

If you had told me a few years ago
that incorporating fasting into my lifestyle could help protect
against various neurodegenerative disorders,
I would have thought you were quite mad.

If you had told me that fasting could positively impact
my happiness, creativity, and personal evolution,
I would have been *certain* you were mad.

However, when we look at how fasting interacts with the brain,
it becomes apparent that there is *much* more to it than just fat loss.

CHALLENGING THE PLASTIC BRAIN

Your mind isn't magic.

It's a moist computer you can program.

- SCOTT ADAMS

Were you ever told that drinking alcohol would kill brain cells *forever*? There *are* many reasons to avoid alcohol, but this particular one may just be a tall tale that Mother relied on to stop us from drinking all night.

The brain can develop and heal by forming new connections throughout our lives. We refer to this as *neuroplasticity*.

Neuroplasticity is the brain's ability to develop and grow throughout life in response to new situations or changes in the environment. For many years, scientists believed that we went through a *critical period* during childhood in which our brain was sponge-like and receptive to learning. After this period, they told us; we set our brain up for life and learning something became much harder. This is an excuse that I, and I'm sure countless others, have used to put off learning something new. However, there has been a paradigm shift in recent times. The current consensus is that the brain can change all the way until we finish this journey we call life. Many disgruntled people bemoan the fact that they did not learn a language or play the violin when they were younger. But in reality, it is *never* too late to learn. When we encounter novel experiences or sensory stimulation, it leaves an *imprint* of sorts on the brain. And whether we can utilise that imprint for learning depends on how *plastic** the brain is. Though it may not seem like it, the brain is reacting to everything going on around us. Contrary to what we believed, and to what many distressed mothers across the globe have said in the past, the brain is *malleable* and able to develop according to our environment and experiences.

Neuroplasticity refers to the flexibility of existing neurons† in the brain to adapt. Neurogenesis refers to the *birth* of new neurons. All throughout life new neurons are born in special parts of the brain, which contribute to learning, memory, and happiness. If we look at the physical size of the brain in neurodegenerative disorders and depression, it is smaller than average because it has *lost* neurons. Neuroplasticity and neurogenesis keep the brain strong and growing.

These are processes integral to our survival. To stimulate them, we will need some resources. A protein called brain-derived neurotrophic factor (BDNF), also known as the *master molecule*, mediates neuroplasticity and neurogenesis. In poetic terms, BDNF is a fertiliser for the brain, allowing it to develop and grow. Methods of enhancing BDNF include more exercise, more sunlight and more sleep. But what if I told you that more *fasting* also stimulates BDNF?

Let's consider Zug in the natural environment in which he evolved. It is challenging. Food is scarce, competition is high, and the hazards are many. Such an environment demands survival adaptations. Zug needs to process information from the environment, such as sights, sounds, and smells, and store it in memory ready for recall. He also

---

*Plastic meaning malleable and able to adapt and change to the environment.

†*Neurons* (also known as nerve cells) are the fundamental units of the brain and nervous system. They are responsible for receiving sensory input from the external world, for sending motor commands to our muscles, and for transforming and relaying the electrical signals at every step in between. Essentially, neurons define who we are as people.

needs to be alert and ready to move. Therefore, he needs BDNF because of the positive role it plays in memory, learning, energy expenditure and fitness levels. The brain produces BDNF when it perceives us to be in a challenging environment. Mother Nature has made it so individuals that find themselves in an environment in which finding food is challenging will be lean, alert and sharp. Because these individuals will *survive*.

But here's the plot twist.

We don't live in a challenging environment anymore, so BDNF lowers and we miss out on the benefits. How can we convince the brain we are in a challenging environment where competition is high and food is scarce? We *could* do lots of fast running. Research has shown that exercise bolsters BDNF production. Even better, we can mimic food scarcity. And the easiest way to do that? *Fasting*.

We don't have to move to a challenging environment to get the benefit of BDNF. All we have to do is incorporate some fasting into our lifestyle. Research on both animals and humans shows this, and the growing scientific consensus is that fasting stimulates BDNF production.

Let's take a deep dive into how fasting and BDNF positively influence our brain health, happiness, and personal evolution.

POWERFUL PEAS, BRAIN CONTROLLERS, AND ENERGETIC HARMONY

Any man could, if he were so inclined,
be the sculptor of his own brain.

- SANTIAGO RAMON Y CAJAL

Mice lacking BDNF are prone to developing obesity, insulin resistance, and anxiety disorders. When researchers inject mice with BDNF, they eat less and move more.

In humans, there is a robust association between low BDNF and the prevalence of both obesity and type 2 diabetes. Researchers have shown that an inherited BDNF deficiency can lead to severe obesity. In fact, scientists now identify stimulating BDNF as a potential therapeutic target for combatting the various facets of metabolic syndrome[*].

But *why* is this?

Scientific circles recognise the important role that BDNF plays in managing the energy balance. To better understand just why this is, we must consider the role that BDNF plays in strengthening the brain. To be specific, within the *hypothalamus*.

The pea-sized hypothalamus is a perfect demonstration of the popular mantra: it's not the size that counts; It's how you use it. Although it accounts for less than *one percent* of the brain, we cannot

[*]Which includes obesity and type 2 diabetes.

underestimate how important the hypothalamus is. Among many other functions, it regulates the release of hormones and guides our emotional and sexual behaviour. The pea-sized powerhouse governs almost everything we do. What we will focus on in this section is how the hypothalamus regulates the energy balance.

Researchers from Tufts University School of Medicine in Boston found that deleting BDNF within the mice hypothalamus increased food intake, reduced activity and led to obesity. In contrast, researchers from the Minnesota Obesity Center injected BDNF into the hypothalamus of mice and observed the opposite effect: decreased food intake and an elevated rate of energy expenditure.

The hypothalamus is like the *controller*. It regulates our energy balance by influencing both our intake of energy and our output. Our friend leptin sends the satisfaction signal to the hypothalamus. When the brain controller operates with ample resources, leptin sensitivity increases and the satisfaction signal is strong, thus helping to regulate appetite. In addition, the pea-sized controller can activate various mechanisms that encourage movement, raise metabolic rate and increase thermogenesis*: all factors that elevate the total rate of energy expenditure and make the energy balance easier to manage.

Brain studies have revealed that hypothalamic function is *compromised* in obesity. The controller has become ineffective, losing control of the energy balance and allowing the vicious cycle to take hold.

You can't plug an ancient controller into a new system and expect optimal performance. Imagine trying to play the latest state-of-the-art game with a controller that only has four buttons. It will not end well. We need to upgrade our controller according to our environment to maintain a healthy balance. BDNF and the resulting plasticity help us do this.

---

* The generation of body heat.

Many claim that fasting can lead to binge eating or even the onset of eating disorders. However, by stimulating BDNF, it may well have the opposite effect. Studies show that a *deficiency* in BDNF can trigger binge-eating episodes and be a strong predictor of weight gain. Research has established an association between low levels of BDNF and eating disorders such as Anorexia Nervosa and Bulimia Nervosa. It is important to note that this does not mean that a lack of BDNF is the root *cause* of these conditions. Eating disorders are complex matters in which there are a multitude of factors at play. They also depend on genetics. Therefore, the main component will always be bio-individuality, but it is still interesting information to marinate on.

AQUATIC STALLIONS, TAXI DRIVERS, AND TELLING STORIES

Learn to use the knowledge of the past and you will look like a genius,
even when you are really just a clever borrower

- ROBERT GREENE

To understand the power of BDNF, we must consider the hippocampus. The word hippocampus comes from the ancient Greek *hippokampus*, which means seahorse. I assume they named it so because of its resemblance to the aquatic stallion. It's all about learning, memory and decision making.

Let's take Henry Molaison as an example. Often referred to as patient H.M, Henry suffered from severe seizures. To get rid of these seizures, he underwent surgery to remove his hippocampus. And the results have ingrained Mr. Molaison in neuroscience folklore. The procedure worked. To an extent. Henry's seizures became less intense and frequent. But there *was* a major downside. He could recall memories from before the surgery, but was incapable of forming new ones. Without his hippocampus, he was living in the past. A tragic case, but it has inspired further research in neuroscience which has shed a lot of light on how the hippocampus works. When a person suffers from memory loss, their hippocampus shrinks. Likewise, when we form new memories, the hippocampus expands. A phenomenon that neuroscientists have observed in London taxi drivers. I'm a London native, so I know them well. If you are not familiar, they drive those famous black cabs; they have an incredible knowledge of a complex city, and they are bloody expensive.

Take a map of Barcelona. It resembles a grid and is easy to navigate. Compare that to a map of London, which looks like the result of a child attacking a piece of paper with a pencil. Within the city, there are thousands of small streets and landmarks. That London taxi drivers can memorise how to navigate such a complex city shows the remarkable capacity that human beings have to learn. The training to become a London taxi driver is notoriously hard. Hopefuls have to pass the world famous *Knowledge*; regarded as the world's toughest taxi test. The Knowledge has been compulsory for taxi drivers since 1865, and it requires memorising all of London's streets. Getting ready for it can take between two and four years. How do they know they are ready? When they feel like an atlas of London has been imprinted into their brain. Given what we know about neuroplasticity, it should come as no surprise that the brain of the taxi driver experiences some profound developments. In the year 2000, Irish neuroscientist Eleanor Maguire found that London taxi drivers had larger than average hippocampi. The reason for this? Their intense training. Learning and storing all of this information expanded the hippocampus. Plasticity in motion.

The hippocampus operates like an information filter. It encodes and stores information according to what it is most useful. Likewise, it is also responsible for how we express this stored information according to the situation. Everyone has a lot of information in their head. To use it to best effect, we have to be selective and use what we need at the right time. This is known as *dynamic* and *flexible* thinking.

For example, let's imagine that you are hosting a dinner party. You have three types of wine: red, white, and rosé. The guests have different preferences. You know that Cassandra loves a good Sauvignon Blanc, whereas Dave does not go near any kind of white wine since that night in Greece. Pouring white wine for everyone, therefore, makes little sense. Instead, you take the information you know and apply it to the situation. You pour Cassandra a glass of your finest New Zealand Sauvignon, while offering Dave a Merlot and sharing a laugh about his infamous white-wine fuelled escapades in Mykonos. The ability to recall stored information and apply it to the situation is the hippocampus in action. A strong hippocampus regulates dynamic and flexible thinking; it can adapt and react to a broad range of circumstances. Likewise, it plays a key role in effective decision making. But what if I told you that strengthening the cerebral seahorse could also enhance your imagination, creativity, social skills, and ability to forgive?

Creativity requires combining existing mental representations to create novel ideas and ways of thinking. In 2013, neuroscientist Melissa Duff and her team at the University of Iowa discovered that the hippocampus may play an important role in creative thinking. They took a group of patients with damage to the hippocampus and a control group of participants with no brain damage and compared their performance on various creative tasks. On one of these tasks, the researchers presented the two groups with an oval shape and asked them to draw a picture with it. The researchers encouraged them to add new ideas and make the picture tell the most interesting and exciting story they could imagine. One participant from the control group made the oval into a giant hot-air balloon that took people for rides above a city. Another participant from the same group used the oval as part of a golf course that included a clubhouse, a sports truck, and even Tiger Woods with his caddy. In contrast, the group with damage to the hippocampus could not create such vivid scenarios. One participant used the oval as an egg with a chicken above it.

Another added legs to the oval to make a bug. Their average creative score was much lower than the control group.

The hippocampus allows us to use stored information in a flexible and dynamic way. Therefore, it governs creative thinking, which is the foundation of *storytelling*. Stories have played a crucial role in our evolution, and storytelling is part of our innate design. Stories transmit messages and information. They are the best way to explain complex concepts as they are easy to remember. And they have the power to evoke a broad range of emotions. Without stories, where would we be? Consider our prehistoric friend. Imagine Zug discovered a threat and wanted to warn the tribe. The best warning would be to tell a story that painted a vivid picture of the situation and evoked emotion. To do so, he would need to call on his stored memories and be creative with them, which would require a strong hippocampus. This cerebral seahorse is also responsible for feeling *empathy*, an integral part of bonding and love. Much like creativity, empathy requires combining various memories and imagining new scenarios. A dynamic hippocampus allows you to put yourself in someone else's shoes. And in the modern world, this can be a *superpower*.

Another way in which the hippocampus influences our behaviour is the role it plays in character judgement. People with a damaged hippocampus are more likely to hold grudges, and less likely to forgive or change their opinions of someone. Even when they see them do something positive. Those with a healthy hippocampus are more open to forgiving a person and changing their judgement according to current behaviour. Holding grudges and being bitter has no place in our everyday life. As Gandhi said, the weak can never forgive; forgiveness is the attribute of the strong. Not letting go holds us back. Forgiveness is the key to happiness, and everything comes from it. Without it, there is no love. When you allow yourself to forgive, you allow yourself to grow.

The hippocampus keeps our thinking and learning *dynamic*. It allows us to adapt, evolve, and grow as a person. In this sense, it may share more similar qualities with the seahorse than just its appearance. When I was younger, the seahorse seemed ordinary to me. Just another thing in the sea, distracting me from my video games. But now that I'm much older, my perception has evolved. The sea horse is a fascinating creature. I mean this in the nicest way possible, but it doesn't look like it belongs in the sea. It has a backbone, a neck, but no stomach. Without a stomach, it has to keep eating. But because of the threat of predators, it doesn't like to move very far. Therefore, it has developed amazing eyesight to both find food and detect predators. You would be forgiven for thinking Mother Nature did not design the seahorse to be in the sea, but it has learnt from and adapted to the environment and thrived. A healthy hippocampus helps us to do the same: learn, adapt, and *thrive*.

So why am I talking about this seahorse shaped superhero with such passion?

The reason that fasting is important regarding the hippocampus is because this area of the brain has the highest demand for BDNF than any other part. It also has the highest level of neurogenesis, given that it deciphers information and creates new memories. In fact, it is one of the few places in the brain that generates new neurons throughout the entire course of life. Therefore, the hippocampus needs plenty of brain fertiliser, and this tells us how much of an influence BDNF has on how we learn. But it does so much more. BDNF helps us to tell better stories and makes us more creative and more empathetic. It also governs how we behave, how we forgive, and therefore how much love we let into our lives. This is the *master molecule*. And fasting provides it.

As we will see in the next section, BDNF may also play a role in combatting addiction and leaving bad habits behind.

POSITIVE CHAIN REACTIONS, ANXIOUS ALMONDS, AND PUBLIC SPEAKING

Today I escaped anxiety.
Or no, I discarded it, because it was within me,
in my own perceptions - not outside.

- MARCUS AURELIUS

A lack of BDNF can exacerbate addictive and anxiety-like patterns of behaviour. Researchers from the Medical University of South Carolina found that infusing the rodent brain with BDNF prevented cocaine seeking behaviour. People with an alcohol dependency have less BDNF than those who do not have one. Recall what we know about neuroplasticity and neurogenesis, and we see BDNF playing a crucial role in cultivating positive behavioural patterns.

Although it is controversial and perhaps even offensive to those struggling with addictive substances, some argue that it is possible to become *addicted* to food. Food addiction is debatable, but we can easily develop an emotional *dependence* on food. Emotional eating is a common behavioural pattern that research associates with the prevalence of obesity and failure to maintain weight loss.

Mastering the art of fasting liberates us from emotional dependency on food. Let's not forget; it requires *discipline* to fast. Fasting is an art form of resisting temptation, and practicing self-control in one area of life can benefit several others. In a study analysing the significance of self-control, Angela Duckworth, a renowned psychologist and science author, writes:

The capacity to govern ourselves effectively in the face of temptation has profound benefits across every major domain of life functioning.

Implementing fasting starts a contagious chain reaction of self control and discipline. Before you know it, this level of mastery over your desires will infiltrate several other areas of life. In a world full of unhealthy distractions, a robust standard of self-control is *invaluable*. Fasting is Mother Nature's way of helping us to leave our destructive habits and dependencies behind, allowing us to create positive patterns of behaviour and thus prolong our survival. Fasting opens us up to the prospect of change and to embrace new patterns of thought and behaviour that can help us evolve into the best version of ourselves. However, to embrace change, we need to first let go of *fear*, and this brings us to a fascinating place. Austria, to be exact. Researchers from the Medical University of Innsbruck found that mice who were fasting experienced less fear than fed mice because of altered brain activity in the *amygdala*.

The name amygdala comes from the Greek word *amygdale*, which means almond, and it sits just in front of the seahorse. When brain experts think of the Amygdala, fear and the fear of fear, or anxiety, come to mind. If you were to press them for a more specific analysis, they would tell you that the amygdala learns and stores fear and processes anxious emotional states.

Researchers from the University College London observed participants playing the Ms. Pac-Man-from-hell video game while in a brain scanner. In the game, a dot pursues players in a maze. If it catches them, they get shocked*. When participants were safe, the

---

*The shock was part of the psychological experiment. Not the original game.

amygdala was quiet. However, activity in the amygdala increased as the dot got closer. The strength of the shock also played a role. If the proposed shock was strong, then the amygdala would activate earlier and to a greater degree.

The amygdala is a tricky customer, but can fasting help to control it?

Researchers from Peking University in China found that participants who were fasting experienced *less* fear than those who were not. They concluded that fasting enhanced *fear extinction*, which is learning that something is not scary anymore. Even six months on from the original study, the fear had not returned. Not only did fasting help to extinguish fear, but it prevented the fear from resurfacing. We don't forget that something is scary; rather, we learn that we need not be afraid any longer. This is what we mean by fear extinction. Fasting enhances fear extinction and prevents the return of fear. This suggests that the amygdala is communicating with the hippocampus; the almond tells the seahorse that it no longer needs to associate fear with certain memories. This helps us to grow and continue with our personal evolution. For Zug, this was essential for survival. It is also essential for *our* survival in the third millennium because a dysfunctional amygdala develops fears around things that need not scare us. It heightens anxiety, makes us indecisive, and stops us from doing what we want to do and becoming who we are. Getting control of the amygdala is key, and the data suggests that fasting can help us with this.

All very fascinating, and I know what you're thinking.

The evolutionary context.

For the hunter-gatherer, the ability to overcome fear and anxiety would have been vital during periods of food scarcity. If our ancestors allowed fear to consume them, then they could not leave the cave and brave the elements to find food. If they weren't able to leave the cave, they weren't able to *survive*. And we would not be here today.

Fasting brings out the best in us. When you break it down, there can be no other way.

Imagine if fear and anxiety overcame our prehistoric chum Zug each time he left the cave to find food. He would not have lasted very long. Fasting allowed Zug to shake off his anxieties and face his fears. With an empty stomach and his life on the line, Zug would not have had the time nor energy to spend on worry. Not on his love life or whether the others back at the cave thought he was cool or not. Survival was the priority.

Fasting is Mother Nature's way of sitting us down and telling us: *don't sweat the small stuff. Life's too short.*

There is no time for fear or anxiety when survival is in the balance. Harnessing the power to overcome fear and anxiety got us where we are today as a species.

Scared about that presentation you have to give?

Is there a big meeting or sales pitch coming up?

Nervous about going to the gym for the first time?

Perhaps the remedy for our most common fears is a lot more accessible than we thought.

In fact, it turns out we had it at our disposal all along.

The best time to give the speech could be deep into a fast.

Zug and our ancestors would have likely faced endless opportunities to give into fear, self-pity or a broad range of negative emotions that would hold them back. However, that they refused to do so is the reason we are here today. They have left us with a set of innate tools that can help us engineer the very best version of ourselves. Emulating authentic patterns of human behaviour allows us to access these tools and *thrive*, so let us not pass up the opportunity.

MENTAL HEALTH AND THE CEREBRAL ECOSYSTEM

Among other things, neuroplasticity means that emotions such as
happiness and compassion can be cultivated in much the same way
that a person can learn through repetition
to play golf and basketball or master a musical instrument,
and that such practice changes the activity
and physical aspects of specific brain areas.

- ANDREW WEIL

Imagine our friend Zug, struggling to find his next meal and protect the tribe. Fighting death and disease every single day. Life is not easy. Now imagine his reaction when you tell him that there is a time and a place where humans have medicine and virtually infinite food. But everyone is depressed. The recent rapid rise in depression appears like a crisis. Although the stigma towards mental health has eased in recent years, the fact remains that we face a colossal challenge. Global antidepressant use is increasing, and many of these medications work by elevating levels of BDNF.

Today we have everything we need, so what could go wrong? Perhaps it's because we are neglecting to emulate authentic patterns of human behaviour. Although there are some who claim that the rise in depression is because of some doctors diagnosing patients when they are just distressed or unhappy, there is an uncomfortable truth that is *not* up for debate: suicide is on the rise.

The World Health Organization reports that worldwide suicide rates have increased by 60% in the last 45 years, and it is now among the three leading causes of death for males and females aged between 15 and 44.

The numbers are tragic, but they do not lie.

The good news is that BDNF and brain plasticity could play a crucial role in preventing depression and regulating mental health. In a study published in the journal *Pharmacology Biochemistry and Behavior*, researchers from Regeneron, a leading biotechnology company, found a strong association with a BDNF deficiency and suicide and suicidal tendencies.

When we consult the data, it presents a well-established link between BDNF and depression, with scientists regarding low levels of BDNF as an important biomarker for several psychiatric disorders, including depression. The growing consensus is that BDNF has a very important role to play.

To further clarify this role, Dr. Yogesh Dwivedi, a decorated researcher who specialises in the neurological basis of depression and suicide, reviewed the critical evidence. In his findings, which the *Journal of Neuropsychiatric Disease and Treatment* published, Doctor Dwivedi concluded:

Several preclinical and clinical observations indicate that depression may be associated with the inability of neural systems to exhibit adaptive plasticity. Given the role of BDNF and its cognate receptors in neural and structural plasticity, and that depression and antidepressants exert opposite actions on BDNF and TrkB expression and functions, it is apparent that BDNF signaling may be crucial in the pathophysiology of depression and in the mechanism of action of antidepressants.

A brain that lacks plasticity and cannot develop according to the living experience is at risk of stagnating and developing depressive symptoms. And a brain deficient in BDNF is just that: a brain unable to change and develop according to the environmental stimuli, which will be detrimental to the human psyche.

Take-home message: brains that lack plasticity are at a very high risk of developing depression, and to cultivate plasticity, we need ample reserves of BDNF. Incorporating fasting ensures that we are never running short.

Another fasting-induced factor that may play a significant role in mental health is *orexin*.

If you recall from earlier on in the book, orexin is the hormone responsible for wakefulness that keeps us feeling alert and energetic. You will also recall that fasting stimulates orexin activity. Scientists from the UCLA found that people who were laughing or feeling excited had higher levels of orexin compared to when they were frustrated or sad. The study also found that levels of orexin were low in subjects who had attempted suicide in the past.

How could orexin, the hormone that regulates wakefulness, breed positivity? Well, it makes us feel alert and energetic, and it is a lot easier to be negative when we are sitting around feeling lethargic doing nothing. In fact, many psychologists agree that idleness and inactivity are powerful contributing factors in depression. When we are on our toes and feeling focused, sensations synonymous with stimulated orexin activity, it is much more straightforward to be proactive and facilitate positivity.

Mental health is a complex issue governed by a multitude of factors, and I do not wish to present fasting as a *cure-all* in such a complex and tragic department. But the data is interesting, and it merits discussion. Fasting and mental health appear to be unrelated. But the fact that fasting stimulates BDNF expression, and to a lesser extent orexin production, suggests that incorporating fasting *could* be a cultivator of a healthy mental ecosystem.

SPIRITUALITY, THE BIG PICTURE, AND FLOW

An overactive ego is a tyrant.

- MICHAEL POLLAN

In Jainism and Buddhism, fasting is often practised alongside meditation. Followers of Jainism fast on specific days of the lunar cycle, whereas in Buddhism, they often practise fasting daily. In the thirteen ascetic* practices developed by Buddha, eating one meal a day is number five, also known as Ekāsanika.

The relationship between fasting and meditation in the realm of spirituality and religion is undeniable, and when we consider what is happening in the brain, we see that this connection is no coincidence either.

We can divide the brain into two large-scale networks: the Attention Network and the Default Mode Network (DMN). There are two subsystems within the attention network: the salience network and the executive network. These structures all play a part in focusing on a task. We begin by mind-wandering, which is the domain of the DMN. The salience network then makes us aware of relevant stimuli, after which the executive network shifts our attention to what needs to be done and then the focus can begin.

---

*an adjective relating to *asceticism*, the doctrine that one can reach a high spiritual state through the practice of extreme self-discipline and abstention from indulgence.

Essentially, when we are engaged, the attention network is engaged. The DMN, however, lights up when we *disengage*. It is probably the strongest candidate in the brain for what you might call the biological home of the ego.

Have you ever lied down for a few minutes of peace, only for your mind to wander through all kinds of hypothetical scenarios and worries? The original plan was to relax, but you ended up worrying about whether Karen from accounts likes your new trousers or if she just thinks you're a buffoon. It is when we enter this internal, imaginative, mental time-travelling state that the DMN comes to life, and the ego takes control.

When we allow the ego to take over, it can limit the lived experience, because it views life through a narrow lens. Temporarily separating from the ego allows us to see the bigger picture and to gain clarity and perspective. If we look at what happens in the brain during psychedelic experiences, in particular with psilocybin-containing mushrooms, the DMN disintegrates, allowing a person to escape their thoughts and see the bigger picture. This experience is like the overview effect, which astronauts experience when they look at the earth from a distance and realise just how insignificant their problems really are.

Leaving the DMN allows us to put things into perspective and to have our own personal overview effect moment, where we realise that perhaps things aren't so bad after all. To see the bigger picture, to clarify what is important, and to keep the ego under control is integral to living a life rich in happiness and fulfillment.

The DMN is responsible for mental time travel. It seems to be most active when we are thinking about the past or the future, and it also lights up when we worry about how other people perceive us. Today, more and more people are becoming trapped in their own thoughts and worrying about what others think of them. Straying from authentic patterns of human behaviour has allowed the DMN to run riot, and this is perhaps why meditation has become so popular in mainstream culture, as it offers a momentary break from the mental gymnastics. Researchers from Emory University took fourteen meditation practitioners and had them perform breath-focused meditation while undergoing fMRI scanning. They instructed the participants to press a button whenever they felt as if their mind was wandering before they returned to focus on their breathing. The researchers found that activity within certain areas of the DMN was higher when participants pressed this button. Likewise, when the participants became more immersed in the practice of meditation, activity within these same areas of the DMN appeared to decrease. When activity in the DMN diminishes, we feel more *present*. And feeling present is not only the key to successful meditation but also for making the most out of life and optimising our happiness. Centering ourselves is also a blessing for productivity, because a less active DMN makes it a lot easier to enter *flow states*.

If you are familiar with Mihaly Csikszentmihalyi's work, then you will already know what flow states are. If you are not, then I would highly recommend his excellent book *Flow: the classic work on how to achieve happiness*. In the meantime, I will offer a little insight. Flow states are essentially the pinnacle of concentration, like being *in the zone*. A person can consider themselves in a flow state when they are so immersed in a certain task or activity that they almost lose track of time.

Flow means less time travel and more focus, which is desirable, not only for productivity but for happiness too. It's very hard to worry about all the insignificant matters of life when you are deep in focus. When I'm fully concentrated on a task, Karen and her thoughts (or lack thereof) regarding my new trousers do not cross my mind.

Therefore, reducing DMN activity can be both therapeutic and productive. Meditation is one method of escaping the clutches of the DMN, but I propose that *fasting* has a similar effect. Researchers from Aachen University in Germany scanned the brains of subjects who had been fasting for fifteen hours and found that there was less activity in the DMN compared to participants who were not fasting. The difference was not huge by any means, but fifteen hours is a relatively short fast, and the researchers concluded that fasting for longer has the potential to amplify this trend.

Don't forget that the brain uses energy. When there is an ample supply of glucose, it will use glucose. However, when the glucose runs out, it will have to find another fuel source, and the breakdown of fat supplies this through the release of ketone bodies. One theory is that ketone bodies preferentially power the attention network as it would be more efficient in finding food and ensuring survival.

To help explain why fasting, focus and flow states go hand in hand, let's take our chum Zug as an example.

Zug has not eaten in a while. If Zug was busy worrying about his shortcomings or whether Skoba thought he was a worthy mate, then he would struggle to find food in the challenging environment. Food scarcity demanded that Zug be present and engaged, so naturally, the DMN would not get a look in during such times.

Flow states are the perfect accompaniment to periods of food scarcity. If Zug has not eaten for a while, then survival and Mother Nature demand that he concentrates, as his life is at risk. This is in stark contrast to today. For example, when Mo feels hungry, he can buy more food with ease. In the modern world, finding food requires very little concentration. In fact, you may even see people a million miles away from flow, ordering their food while simultaneously paying attention to something on their phone. Not very authentic patterns of human behaviour methinks.

Modern food availability represents an evolutionary millisecond.

For most of our time on earth, we had to find food with our own hands, so being able to focus during periods of food scarcity was *essential*.

If Zug's survival is on the line while he is chasing a gazelle or climbing a tall tree for some fruit, then Mother Nature will demand that his levels of concentration are at full capacity. Being able to enter flow states during periods of food scarcity is an innate survival mechanism.

Throughout most of our evolution, there would have been little opportunity to get lost mind-wandering in the DMN. Today, however, we seem to have an awful lot of downtime, so there is more space for the mind to wander, and unfortunately, it can often lead to negative places.

Fasting and flow states are another example of how we can use an ancient survival adaptation to *thrive* in the third millennium. We don't need to hunt or gather our food, so we can instead utilise fasting to shift into flow states and supercharge our productivity and happiness.

Many people report feeling happier, more productive and mentally sharper while fasting, and perhaps this is because of reduced activity in the DMN and a clearer pathway into flow states.

Besides enhancing our concentration, fasting also allows us to step back and see the big picture.

In a world full of distractions, this could prove *invaluable*.

GREEK WISDOM, NAKED APPLES, AND STAYING STRONGER FOR LONGER

Fasting cleanses the soul, raises the mind,
subjects one's flesh to the spirit, renders the heart contrite and humble,
scatters the clouds of concupiscence, quenches the fire of lust,
and kindles the true light of chastity.
Enter again into yourself.

- AUGUSTINE OF HIPPO

Few know of this, but the Ancient Greeks used fasting to treat epilepsy in children as far back as 500 BC. When the most prolific thinkers in history were delivering timeless nuggets of wisdom, they were also exploring the therapeutic use of fasting. In modern times, making children fast is questionable, so to circumvent this problem, doctors developed the ketogenic diet which mimics the effects of fasting on seizure control in the 1920s as a treatment for epilepsy. Although the therapeutic use of the ketogenic diet and fasting for treating epilepsy began to die down when a wide range of pharmaceutical drugs became available from 1940 onwards, recent years have seen these more traditional methods enjoy a huge surge in popularity. Ketone bodies are the crucial component here. A growing amount of data shows that ketones can alter neuronal activity that helps to protect against seizures, hence why fasting and the ketogenic diet are so useful in treating epilepsy. But there could be more to them.

Ketones may have other neuroprotective properties, as a growing body of emerging research suggests that the ketogenic diet can help to treat disorders such as Alzheimers and Parkinsons. The data is promising but not conclusive. However, scientists agree that ketone bodies can protect against various neurodegenerative disorders because they reduce oxidative stress by keeping the free radical *cowboys* under control. Fasting and using ketone bodies for fuel increases metabolic flexibility and decreases oxidative stress. In longevity, this is significant because too much oxidative stress speeds up the ageing process.

Despite only weighing around two percent of the body, the brain requires up to twenty percent of the energy supply, making it especially vulnerable to oxidative damage. Excessive oxidative stress can cause cellular damage and impair the DNA repair system, both key factors in speeding up the ageing process and developing neurodegenerative disorders.

One characteristic of Alzheimer's disease is the buildup of toxic amyloid plaques in the brain, which destroy synaptic connections[*]. Research shows that oxidative stress plays a critical role in the initiation and progression of Alzheimers because it enhances the production of these amyloid plaques. Scientists also consider oxidative stress to be one of the major mechanisms underlying Parkinson's disease. Therefore, correcting oxidative imbalance and reducing oxidative stress has become an area of great interest in the fields of neuroscience and longevity. This has resulted in antioxidant therapy being suggested to prevent and treat neurodegenerative disorders, but researchers are yet to find an effective formula.

---

[*]Each neuron may be connected to up to 10,000 other neurons, passing signals to each other via as many as 1,000 trillion synaptic connections. These connections are responsible for the transfer of information and retrieval of memories. Hence why their destruction can lead to memory loss.

In the meantime, fasting can offer protection for our brains while we continue the search for answers. Fasting is not a panacea, but it does limit free radicals and reduce oxidative stress. It is also very easy to incorporate and maintain, so it is a good place to start in strengthening our cerebral defences. Reducing oxidative stress can have massive implications for the optimisation of overall health and longevity. To save paper, and to not bore you, I shall communicate this point through a digestible diagram.

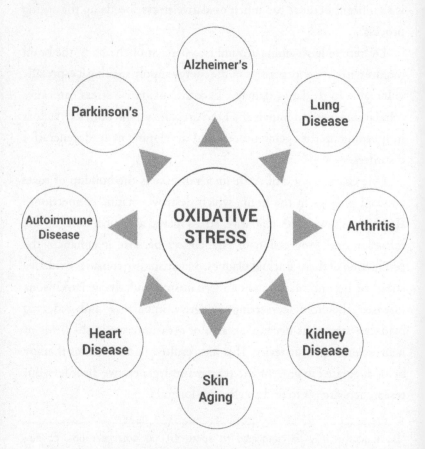

As you can see, oxidative stress is best avoided. Fasting helps us to steer clear.

Excessive oxidative stress will also accelerate the aging process on an *aesthetic* level. When free radicals are too many and oxidative stress occurs, our skin pays a high price. It can dry out, wrinkle and lose its vigor, which is perhaps why those with an unhealthy lifestyle often appear to be tired and have weathered skin. Scientists agree that the skin is a prime target of oxidative stress, as it possesses a very large surface area and several physiological components susceptible to the effects of oxidative damage, such as DNA and proteins. A helpful way to understand how oxidative stress affects the skin and how it operates is to imagine an *apple*.

Yes, an apple.

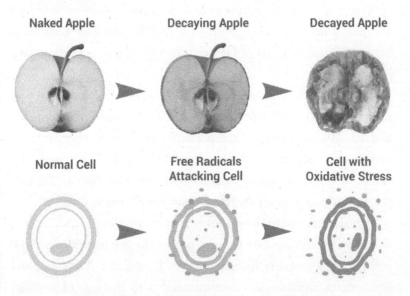

The naked apple dries out and withers away when exposed to oxidative damage with poor defences in place. A similar effect happens in the cells, leading to premature ageing and even disease.

We *can* increase antioxidant intake through diet, but the optimal strategy would be to address the danger at the source. Implementing certain lifestyle changes that help to prevent the buildup of free radicals and reduce exposure to oxidative stress is a wise strategy.

This allows us to tackle the root of the problem. Adding things here and there may paper over the cracks but they won't be much help in the long run.

Fasting is an excellent method of reducing oxidative stress, which could help to explain why so many people often report that their skin seems to appear more vibrant and healthy after they embrace the fasting lifestyle.

Another topic we discussed before was how fasting elevates growth hormone production.

When we think of growth hormone, the main things that come to mind is preserving or building muscle mass, but healthy levels of GH also play a key role in longevity. Many studies show an association between declining levels of GH and the typical effects of the ageing process.

The various consequences of a GH deficiency reflect its importance in the ageing process, such as increased fat mass, decreased muscle and strength, decreased exercise performance, decreased bone mineral density, increased risk of fracture, and dry skin. GH deficiency also comes with several various psychological problems that can decrease the overall quality of life such as fatigue, depression and anxiety.

It is also important to remember that *muscle* plays a crucial role in longevity. Preserving muscle mass, one of the key functions of GH, will optimise mobility throughout life. Losing the ability to move has serious psychological consequences, with the loss of mobility cited as one of the leading causes of depression amongst the elderly. Maintaining the capacity for movement will increase the level of enjoyment one can extract from each passing day as they become less young. As Michael McLeod, a researcher on musculoskeletal ageing from the University of Birmingham, concluded in a study that reviewed the role of muscle mass in healthy ageing:

Maintaining physical strength is a key strategy that leads to healthy ageing.

Another reason to thrash some weights around. Strength and mobility are two factors that make becoming less young more enjoyable. Aside from slowing down the ageing process, another fascinating aspect of GH is the role it plays in reproductive health. Clinicians have used GH supplementation in managing both male and female infertility to improve pregnancy rates in poor responders. To construct a brand new human being will require ample amounts of the hormone responsible for growth, which helps to explain the relationship between GH and fertility.

Further studies show that GH can increase libido in both men and women, and there is even strong evidence demonstrating the important role that GH plays in maintaining *male erectile capability*. Growth hormone: the clue is in the name. No growth, no party. Remember, everything links back to Mother Nature's prioritisation of survival during periods of food scarcity and perceived danger.

Boosting GH and reducing oxidative stress with fasting could be key in living stronger for longer.

SUMMARY

Because of the power of neuroplasticity, you can, in fact, reframe your
world and rewire your brain so that you are more objective.
You have the power to see things as they are
so that you can respond thoughtfully, deliberately, and effectively
to everything you experience.

- ELIZABETH THORNTON

Well, that was quite the section, if I say so myself.
Time for a deep breath, a moment of reflection and perhaps a siesta.
Take your time.

I have been saying for many years that I believe fasting possesses benefits which transcend the realm of weight loss. And now that you know a little more of how fasting interacts with the brain, you may share this belief.

Scientists agree that, from a medical perspective, there are several potential therapeutic uses of fasting. If we consider this along with the wealth of data showing the benefits of BDNF, the implications for brain health and longevity could be huge. By stimulating BDNF and reducing oxidative stress, a fasting lifestyle could help to combat memory loss and several neurodegenerative disorders, such as Alzheimer's and Parkinson's. It will also go a long way in enhancing our lived experience, and ensuring that it goes on for as long as possible.

Fasting is therapy. And in more ways than one.

Part Six

FASTING FOR THE FUTURE

The modern person is not just eating more than ever.

They are eating more *often* than ever.

Most diseases in the developed world are diseases of *abundance*,
not of scarcity.

I often hear that fasting is just another tool for losing weight.

This is not necessarily untrue, as it *is* a useful tool to improve body
composition and lose fat.

But only looking at fasting through a weight-loss lens does it
a great disservice. In reality, fasting can offer so much more*.

It is all about adaptations that keep us thriving in the game of life
for as long as possible.

As Charles Darwin alluded to in his *On the Origin of Species*,
the best is not the strongest or the most intelligent.

But the one that is most able to *adapt* to change.

---

*To clarify, when I talk about fasting in this section, I am not referring to fasting
indefinitely. Rather, I refer to a fasting *lifestyle* in which fasting and feeding are
part of a balanced approach.

DIABETES

We're not meant to consume infinite news, infinite porn, infinite food. We live in an era of too much abundance. This is the modern struggle.

- NAVAL RAVIKANT

Prediabetes is the last stop before type 2 diabetes, and its prevalence is rising worldwide. Researchers predict that over 470 million people will be prediabetic within ten years. Seventy percent of those people will develop type 2 diabetes. According to scientists, the key to preventing prediabetes lies in lifestyle changes. Perhaps the best place to start is emulating authentic patterns of human behaviour.

In 2018, Elizabeth Sutton and her team at the Pennington Biomedical Research Center in Louisiana wanted to see if fasting offered any benefits outside of fat loss. They took six men with prediabetes and assigned them to one of two groups. In the first group, they ate within a six-hour window. In the second, a twelve hour window. Participants adhered to the conditions for five weeks before crossing over to the other group for another five weeks. The focus was not on fat loss, and the researchers fed each participant enough to maintain their weight. At the end of the study, fasting had reduced blood pressure, oxidative stress, and appetite. Perhaps the most important development was the improvement in *insulin sensitivity*.

Insulin resistance, as the name suggests, is the body becoming *resistant* to insulin. And it is the main driver of prediabetes. The key to reducing resistance is to increase sensitivity. We need to make peace with insulin. And we can do this with fasting. A fasting lifestyle increases insulin sensitivity and can reverse prediabetes. Reversing prediabetes will prevent type 2 diabetes. And the implications for humanity are *huge*.

Type 2 diabetes is an epidemic growing to cosmic proportions and posing a serious threat to the future of humanity. Across the globe, the number of people with diabetes has risen from 108 million in 1980 to 422 million in 2014. In 2016, diabetes was the direct cause of 1.6 million deaths, and in 2012 high blood sugar caused another 2.2 million deaths. The numbers are overwhelming, and this trend shows no sign of slowing down. Let's stop and think about how far we have come since 1980.

In 1980, the Internet did not exist, and there were no mobile phones, let alone smartphones. Since 1980, extreme poverty has been in sharp decline. In 1980, 1.9 billion people across the world lived in extreme poverty. In 2018, that number is down to 650 million. In 1980, my dad could go to the pub and not worry about making an excuse why he ignored my mother's calls, because no one had a mobile phone. Since 1980, life expectancy across the world has skyrocketed. For example, the average life expectancy of an Ethiopian in 1980 was 43.7 years. In 2015, it has increased to 65 years. Although the world in which we live today is not without its problems, it is a *much* safer place than 40 years ago. According to several metrics, the world in which we live is getting better and better. Yet despite all this, diabetes and obesity have gotten *worse*. How could this have happened?

In 2012, the cost of diabetes in the United States was 245 billion dollars. And this is not including the many prediabetic people who will develop type 2 diabetes. If nothing changes, annual US spending on diabetes in fifteen years will be around 336 billion dollars.

Three hundred and thirty-six billion dollars.

That number is so enormous, it doesn't even make sense anymore. Especially when you consider that type 2 diabetes is *preventable*. If you perform a quick mental analysis of the information, you would conclude that our modern eating habits are not interacting optimally with our physiology. We have reached a stage where we have neglected emulating authentic patterns of human behaviour and we are paying a high price for it. If we do not act, this crisis *will* get worse. The onus is on us to intervene and take action. The ball is in our court. We must focus on *prevention*. What we need is a *game changer*.

First, an important distinction. Type 1 diabetes is an *inability* to produce insulin. Those with type 1 struggle to gain weight and have to take insulin regularly. Fasting lowers insulin, so we do not consider it a treatment for type 1, and it could be very dangerous*. Genetics largely determine type 1, whereas lifestyle factors govern type 2 diabetes. The case of type 2 is the opposite of type 1. In type 2 diabetes, there is *too much* insulin. So much so it leads to insulin resistance.

Chronically elevated levels of insulin will lead to the overflow phenomenon, in which the feedback system becomes flooded, setting in motion the vicious cycle of insulin resistance. When we raise insulin to an unnatural degree, the system cannot cope. Our unnatural living conditions today make this malfunction possible. Consuming hyper-processed sugary foods around the clock means that that insulin stays spiked. And when there is too much insulin, the cells become less receptive to its key. This means that insulin cannot shuttle sugar out of the blood and into the cells for energy. The pancreas† does not receive the signal that energy has entered the cell, so it recognises this as a *lack* of insulin. It thinks that because the energy cannot enter the cell, then it needs *more* insulin. Therefore, the pancreas continues to pump out more insulin. What the body needs is a *break*, not

---

* Anyone with type 1 diabetes must consult their doctor before making changes.
† The pancreas is an organ of the digestive system and plays an essential role in converting food into fuel for the body's cells by producing insulin.

more insulin. Imagine you are trying to talk to someone who has headphones on. You say something, but they don't hear you. All they hear is background noise, so they turn the volume up to cancel it out. The logical thing to do in this situation is to remove their headphones so they can hear you clearly. But what the pancreas does is insist on talking *louder*, so the person with headphones continues to increase the volume, and the signal never gets through. In this situation, the pancreas is like the five-year-old me who thought rolling in coal was a good substitute for having a bath. It means well, but it ends up making the situation worse. What the body needs is to lower levels of insulin to regain its function and reverse the resistance. Producing more insulin has the opposite effect. Increasing insulin only serves to further compound the resistance. And so the vicious cycle begins. What the body needs is a break. What the body needs is *fasting*.

Hormones are all closely connected. And they like a balance. If one plays up, the rest become imbalanced, and chaos ensues. Insulin is one of the most important hormones in the body, and it affects everything. When a person becomes resistant to insulin, other hormones, such as leptin and melatonin, become imbalanced. This wreaks havoc on appetite and sleeping habits, which serves to feed the vicious cycle and speed up the development of type 2 diabetes. But this is not the only risk. Scientists associate high levels of insulin in the blood to obesity, heart disease, and cancer. Once the insulin system becomes compromised, the body panics. Lowering insulin resistance is the key to preventing a broad range of diseases*. And to reverse insulin resistance, we need insulin sensitivity.

Fasting is mother nature's insulin sensitiser. If we don't eat, we cannot raise insulin. For a person struggling with prediabetes, this will be crucial. Lowering insulin will increase insulin sensitivity and help to break out of the vicious cycle. And the best way to lower insulin

---

*Also known as *metabolic syndrome*

is to fast. The mainstream have overlooked the fasting lifestyle, but it could be the key to preventing type 2 diabetes. Did I mention that it is easy to do, it can improve several other areas of life and does not cost a penny? It's a no-brainer, dawg.

Type 2 diabetes is the last stage of a vicious cycle, and scientists are still unsure how to treat it. Emerging research suggests that a fasting lifestyle can help[*].

Jason Fung is a Toronto-based doctor who has inspired many to embrace fasting. His book, *The Obesity Code*, polarised opinions within some circles. But what is not up for debate is the fact that he is on the front-lines treating patients with type 2 diabetes. In many cases, he is giving people their lives back[†]. The British Medical Journal published an example of his work using therapeutic fasting to treat and manage type 2 diabetes.

Three patients with type 2 diabetes did regular twenty-four-hour fasts over a period of several months. At the end of the study, all three patients discontinued their insulin medication, with two of them able to discontinue *all* diabetic medications. They all lost weight and inches off their waist and reported fewer cravings and more energy. And they all agreed that fasting was easy and rather enjoyable. Another crucial element is that, by incorporating fasting, the patients could manage their own diabetes, rather than having to rely on factors outside of their control. This style of approach will be beneficial in reducing the common feelings of helplessness. And as patient 2 said, it made them feel *terrific*. Fasting gave them a new lease of life.

We need more research, but one thing is clear: we have greater control over the diabetes epidemic than we thought. Prevention is within our control, and the key lies in emulating authentic patterns of human behaviour. The easiest place to start is fasting.

---

[*]Anyone with type 2 diabetes must consult their doctor before making changes.
[†]I recommend his second book the *Diabetes Code* for those interested

OBESITY

A fast is better than a bad meal.

- IRISH PROVERB

Telling an obese individual they need to eat less and move more to lose weight is like telling a depressed person all they need to do is to *be happy*. It makes sense, but only at a very basic level. It is a lot easier said than done, and as far as advice goes, it is more or less *worthless*. As the legendary poet Ralph Waldo Emerson once said:

Once you make a decision, the universe conspires to make it happen.

This is one of my favourite quotes, and I often apply it to emphasise why it is important to believe in yourself. I could also apply it to obesity. Once a person gains a significant amount of body fat, their brain, body and the entire world, then conspire to keep hold of it. And to understand why this is, we must consider how our hormones react to us putting on significant amounts of excess fat.

Excessive body fat elevates leptin to levels that can lead to leptin resistance, in which the satisfaction signal struggles to reach its destination and results in an insatiable appetite. As a person eats more and gains more weight, they struggle to feel satisfied from food, so they eat more and gain more weight. Obesity itself is a vicious cycle for various reasons, and a dysfunctional satisfaction signalling system is one of them.

In obesity, leptin is struggling, which is both tragic and paradoxical.

Tragic because we are quick to judge obese individuals and conclude that a lack of willpower led them to this situation. But in reality they could be deep in the throes of a vicious cycle and losing control. It is paradoxical because if a person eats *more*, then they should feel satisfied. However, in obesity, the exact opposite occurs, with obese individuals eating more and gaining more weight yet feeling *less* satisfied. In obese individuals, levels of leptin are very high, which leads one to think small amounts of food would satisfy them. But the large amounts of body fat in obese individuals has raised leptin so much that it floods the feedback system and they become resistant to the satisfaction signal.

I'm sure you have met someone who is overweight yet *never* satisfied with food. We often regard this as simple greed or a lack of willpower, but the situation is a lot more complex and not only the fault of the individual. In obesity, there is a multitude of factors at play.

We do not place enough emphasis on the *vicious* nature of obesity, and how difficult it can be to escape the cycle. Some good news, however, is that fasting can help to sensitize us to the satisfaction signal because it lowers levels of leptin, thus reducing leptin resistance. Research has also identified high levels of leptin as a strong predictor of weight *regain* in obese individuals.

Repairing a damaged satisfaction signalling system is key in developing the behavioural patterns necessary to reverse obesity. To escape the vicious cycle, leptin must be under control, and this is where fasting can help.

VICIOUS CYCLES, DRAWING BLANKS, AND SKIPPING BREAKFAST SHOWS

I find television very educating.

Every time somebody turns on the set,

I go into the other room and read a book.

- GROUCHO MARX

An additional problem that we face regarding the obesity crisis is a lack of *ideas*.

Obesity rates have been rising worldwide since 1980, with the trend experiencing a sharp increase in recent years. Much like with type 2 diabetes, it shows no signs of slowing down soon. In the United States, the estimated annual health care cost of obesity-related illnesses amounts to a staggering 190 billion dollars. In terms of cost, obesity has now overtaken smoking as a public health enemy number one.

If you live in the UK, you will know the NHS is under a great deal of pressure. Between 2014 and 2015, the NHS spent six billion pounds on overweight and obesity related ill-health, and these numbers continue to rise. In a study looking at projected obesity trends that respected medical journal *The Lancet* published, lead author Claire Wang paints a bleak picture for the future if nothing changes:

The combined medical costs associated with treatment of these preventable diseases (stemming from obesity) are estimated to increase by $48-66 billion/year in the USA and by £1·9-2 billion/year in the UK by 2030. Hence, effective policies to promote healthier weight also have economic benefits.

These numbers are shocking. Even more so when we consider the fact that obesity, as Claire Wang states in her analysis, is *preventable*.

The health risks associated with obesity are many. Cancer, diabetes, hypertension, stroke, liver disease, heart disease, sleep apnea, and chronic back pain to name a few. However, something that we forget is the impact obesity has on *mental* health. Getting caught in the unforgiving cycle of obesity can make a person feel helpless, which explains why research has linked obesity with depression. Obesity is a vicious cycle not only in terms of physical health, but mental health too, so it is time to take control. It is time to *change the game*.

Our genetic design is not compatible with the modern sedentary lifestyle. Efforts to stem the prevalence of obesity have been ineffective, so we must expand the conversation and explore alternative avenues.

I recall one British breakfast show in which the panel were discussing a new medication called *lorcaserin* that was being touted as a cure for obesity. Lorcaserin is a mild appetite suppressant. Clinical trials have shown that a group using lorcaserin only had a 3.3% difference in weight loss when compared to a placebo group. The weight loss benefit was minor, but there *was* a significant finding from the research: the list of potential side effects including increased risk of heart attacks and depression.

Considering these potential side effects, the minor weight loss effect that lorcaserin has seems trivial. That's not all; you would also have to pay a substantial amount for the privilege. One guest on the panel who was a supposed authority on obesity was full of praise for lorcaserin, even labelling it as the *holy grail*.

This is nonsense.

It is nonsensical and *not* a viable solution. I am opposed to labelling *anything* as a holy grail, but let's be crystal clear here. In the arena of combatting obesity, fasting takes lorcaserin, and any appetite suppressant, to the cleaners every day of the week and twice on Sundays.

Fasting is Mother Nature's appetite suppressant, and it does not come with any negative side effects like depression. In fact, perhaps quite the opposite, as we saw in the last part of the book.

Unlike lorcaserin, fasting is *free*. That this panel of professionals were discussing an expensive medication with harmful side effects before they had considered fasting baffled me. Another reason not to watch television.

This paints a clear picture of the authoritative figures running out of ideas. It also shows that skipping television alongside breakfast is a good idea.

It's time to change the game.

The further we stray from authentic patterns of human behaviour, the more prevalent obesity becomes. Mother Nature equipped us with a powerful toolset, but she has not prepared us for a sedentary lifestyle and calorie dense hyper-palatable foods in abundant availability. Perhaps in a hundred thousand years we will have evolved to navigate this kind of territory experiencing no problems, but right now it is proving to be a challenge. Therefore, the key to preventing and reversing obesity must lie in emulating authentic patterns of human behaviour.

And I believe that fasting is a great place to start.

JIGGLY FAT, SURVIVAL MECHANISMS, AND SAVING LIVES

The majority of people have no understanding of the things
with which they daily meet, nor, when instructed,
do they have any right knowledge of them,
although to themselves they seem to have.

- HERACLITUS

An important component of obesity is *fat oxidation**.

We know that fasting increases the rate of fat oxidation. When we fast, we burn more fat for fuel. But the sceptics will say that this is inconsequential as weight loss depends on the energy balance. The latter part of the scepticism is true, but when we consult the research there is a very strong link between low rates of fat oxidation and obesity.

What is going on here? Could fat oxidation be a potential tool in preventing obesity? Well, here's the thing. It depends on what *type* of fat we are burning. We see body fat as one entity, but it contains several types that all possess different characteristics. It may seem like quite a strange concept at first, but not all the fat that we carry is the same. The two types that we will focus on are subcutaneous fat and visceral fat.

We store subcutaneous fat under our skin with the soft jiggly feel.

---

* Scientific term for burning fat for fuel.

Everyone has subcutaneous fat, and although it is responsible for the *appearance* of obesity, it does not carry the main risk factors.

Visceral fat is not as visible but carries with it most of the risk factors associated with obesity. We store it deep in the abdominal cavity where it wraps around organs such as the heart, liver, kidneys, pancreas, and intestines. We refer to these organs as the *viscera*, which would explain where this fat got its name from.

It's straightforward to tell how much subcutaneous fat someone has because of its strong visual presence. However, visceral fat is not so obvious. Excessive fat storage in the belly area *can* be a sign of visceral fat build up, as can a large waist measurement, but these will not tell the whole story. The most certain way to measure visceral fat is an MRI scan, but this is not a very accessible nor economical procedure. The best thing we can do is ensure that we burn as much visceral fat as possible and reduce the risk of storing it.

Visceral fat is a strong risk factor for type 2 diabetes and heart disease, but the dangers extend far beyond metabolic disorders. Research shows that a high level of visceral fat also increases the risk of dementia and Alzheimer's disease. Visceral fat is devastating and it can tear families apart. The most baffling thing of all? You may not have heard of visceral fat before.

In the health and fitness space, they seldom mention visceral fat. People talk about fat loss *ad nauseam*, but they rarely go into specifics. I am a lover of simplicity and allergic to anything complicated, but I believe this is an important topic to discuss. Many people notice visible fat loss in the abdominal area with fasting, or their waist measurement going down without significant weight loss on the scale. Visceral fat only makes up around ten percent of total body fat. Therefore, one could reduce visceral fat without making big changes to their scale weight. If fasting is burning fat for fuel, could it be prioritising the use of the visceral fat from the abdominal area?

Let's frame this one in an evolutionary context.

Why would we hold on to the most harmful kind of fat that can threaten our livelihood if the brain perceives that we are in danger? The fat that poses the most risk to our health would be the first to go as Mother Nature looks to ensure our survival. When discussing autophagy in part four, we mentioned how fasting triggers survival adaptations that remove as many risks to our life as possible, and perhaps a similar operation happens with fat-burning. Subcutaneous fat, although undesirable, does not pose a threat to our livelihood in the same way that visceral fat does, and it is also rather plentiful. Remember, the brain does not know the exact specifics of the situation; it is perceiving fasting as food scarcity. It does not know when this food scarcity may end, so it would be wise to save the safe and plentiful subcutaneous stores for later. In life, it always makes sense to get rid of harmful or substandard things first. And I posit that fasting has a similar effect on fat.

If Zug was facing a period of food scarcity, it would make sense to prioritise the breakdown of visceral fat for fuel because of its life-threatening nature. Remember, it always links back to survival. Burning harmful fat during food scarcity is Mother Nature's way of reducing risk and increasing our chances of survival.

However, relying on the evolutionary argument alone is not enough, so let's dive deeper.

Researchers from Nanjing University in China found that mice prioritised the breakdown of visceral fat for fuel during a day of fasting. During a period of food scarcity, mice burn the life-threatening visceral fat and save the subcutaneous fat for later. In another Chinese study, this time from the Central South University in the province of Hunan, researchers made a fascinating observation. They found mice prioritised the breakdown of visceral fat during a fast, but when they began the refeeding process, they stored excess energy as *subcutaneous* fat, rather than visceral fat. This led the researchers to conclude that fat tissue has a certain *plasticity** in response to fasting. Fasting triggered a survival adaptation that not only removed visceral fat, but stopped it from coming back too. In mice, fasting destroys visceral fat. The rodent research is crystal clear. But let's see what information we can extract from the human research.

Researchers from Aarhus University Hospital in Denmark observed human volunteers during a seventy-two hour fasting period. They found that fasting stimulates the breakdown of fat in the abdominal area and had a *sparing* effect on subcutaneous fat. The results suggest that fasting triggers a similar response in humans as it does in mice, prioritising the breakdown of harmful visceral fat and saving subcutaneous fat for later. We need more research, but these are promising signs.

There is another potential piece of the visceral puzzle that is worth mentioning. Growth hormone also likes to fight fat. Research has linked a *deficiency* in GH to higher levels of visceral fat. And further studies show that growth hormone therapy, which involves administering GH to those who are deficient, reduces visceral fat. GH stimulates the breakdown of fat for fuel, and it appears to prioritize visceral fat. Fasting stimulates GH production as a survival adaptation to keep us burning fat rather than muscle, adding credence to the idea that fasting promotes the breakdown of life-threatening visceral fat. Scientists regard growth hormone as a champion of longevity. What could be more integral to longevity than burning the visceral fat that threatens our life?

Could fasting remove visceral fat and help to keep it off?

Current research and anecdotal evidence shows promise, and the implications for the obesity crisis could be huge.

---

*the ability to be shaped or moulded according to changes in the environment.

MOVING MORE
WITH JULIA
AND THE AMISH
(*not a sitcom*)

Look to your own means, leave everything that isn't yours alone.
Make use of what material advantages you have,
don't regret the ones you were not allowed.

- EPICTETUS

The various causes underlying obesity are complex, but a lack of physical activity is one that we can all agree on. The further we stray from authentic patterns of human behaviour, the more problems we encounter. As we continue to automate much of our everyday life and disregard our nature, the more inactive we become. The easier we make it to do everything, the harder it becomes to stay active.

Scientists use the term *physical inactivity* to identify people who do not get the recommended level of physical activity, and they estimate around 31% of adults worldwide are physically inactive. In the United States, physical inactivity affects almost half of the population. Researchers have established increasing physical activity as one of the main therapeutic targets for managing obesity. But cajoling obese people to dive straight into an intense exercise program can come with various risks. Exercise triggers a temporary spike in blood pressure. And although for most people this is a beneficial adaptation, for those struggling with obesity it can be precarious as they may already have high blood pressure. Because of excess weight, intense exercise strains the joints of obese individuals and carries the risk of serious injury. Obese people are much more susceptible to heat exhaustion and dehydration because they have more difficulty regulating their body temperature than non-obese people. For those struggling with obesity, intense exercise carries certain risks. I am not, however, saying that we should avoid exercise altogether.

Exercise is beneficial. But it is not the *only* way, and obese individuals should look to introduce it into their lifestyle gradually to reduce the aforementioned risks. Unlike structured exercise that demands intensity, NEAT does not present similar risks in terms of injury. NEAT includes activities such as washing the dishes, walking to work and even bird watching, in which the risk of injury is low (unless you come across an angry bird). Increasing NEAT can also account for a large expenditure of energy for those who are overweight because they have more weight to move around.

Another potential pitfall of instructing obese people to exercise is that of *adherence*.

Exercise is beneficial, but if we consult the research, we see that those struggling with obesity also struggle with adhering to a regular exercise program. In one study published in the *Journal of Eating and Weight Disorders*, researchers from the University of Florence concluded:

Regular physical exercise is a widely accepted means of reducing mortality and improving a number of health outcomes, which is also efficacious in the treatment of obesity. Unfortunately, despite the evidence of favourable short- and long-term effects, the results seem to be affected by a lack of adherence, particularly over the long term

The benefits are clear, but for someone who struggles with obesity, it's difficult to stay consistent with exercise. Compliance with exercise is low, but NEAT has a much higher rate of adherence, because it is *accessible.* Many people only have a small window of time in which to exercise. Maybe they have a family or long working hours, and this is where NEAT steps in, as we can do it *anywhere.*

Julia is adamant that she does not have the time for exercise, and she often cites a lack of time as the reason she is struggling with her weight. She has already incorporated a fasting schedule, but let's look at her typical day and see if she can make any neat modifications to increase her activity levels. The first diagram is what she does now, and the second is how her typical day could look like with more NEAT.

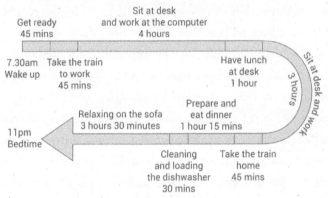

On a typical day, Julia spends a lot of time sitting down and doing very little. Let's see if we can change that.

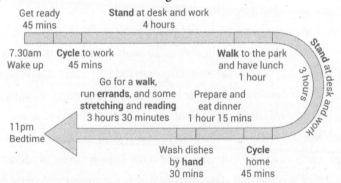

As you can see, Julia has plenty of opportunity to get more active and break out of the vicious cycle. Over time, these small modifications can amount to huge changes. It doesn't just have to be exercise, and it does not require a huge investment of time, effort, or money. Julia has had her mind blown to bits. If we imagine that she is a 5"3" tall 45 year old woman weighing 180 lbs and struggling with obesity, then making these kind of modifications could lead her to lose 25 lbs in three months. And it would go a long way in reversing obesity.

Outside of time, NEAT has another dimension of accessibility. For an obese person, it can be quite intimidating to walk into a gym or an exercise class, and it can confuse knowing where to start. Some people do not have access to a gym in which to take part in structured exercise. However, they can incorporate NEAT with ease. As a bonus, it is free and always will be. I should, however, clarify that we should not consider NEAT as a like-for-like substitution for exercise. Rather it is a substitute for the time that we would otherwise spend doing very little, like watching television for example.

Increasing NEAT is not just about losing weight; it can also reduce the long-term risk of cardiovascular disease and all-cause mortality. One large-scale study from the Karolinska University Hospital in Stockholm, Sweden, followed 3839 patients over the course of 12 and a half years. The researchers found that those who maintained higher levels of NEAT reduced their risk of cardiovascular disease by 27% and all-cause mortality by 30%.

An enormous portion of the population are now spending most of their waking time sitting down. Though it may seem innocuous, it is becoming apparent that large periods of time spent sitting down can be detrimental to our health in the long term. Researchers have linked prolonged periods of time spent sitting down with the prevalence of cardiovascular disease and type 2 diabetes. How many people do you know suffering from back pain because of slouching in front of a screen all day? Sitting down for prolonged periods of time is not an authentic pattern of human behaviour. And with the help of fasting, we can relegate it to the waste bin of history. Given all the technological advances and contraptions available to us, there is no excuse for sitting down all day. If you work at an office and feel trapped, we can change the desk to accommodate a standing position. I did it myself using only books as make-shift platforms to elevate my computer and keyboard. It is always possible. By doing away with so much time spent sitting down, we move closer to optimal health and increasing our levels of NEAT. Two birds; one stone.

The research shows that increasing NEAT is an integral tool in managing obesity and the associated risk factors, yet it is often overlooked. This could be because it just doesn't *feel* like activity. Increasing our daily activity, by walking more for example, doesn't feel like thrashing around the battle ropes like a lunatic. But we cannot underestimate the benefit of increasing NEAT over the long-term.

It all comes back to authentic patterns of human behaviour. Today, we have a plethora of tools and machines that can take care of everyday tasks for us; more jobs that require sitting down for prolonged periods of time; and a reduction in movement. It is clear to see where this is taking us. And it doesn't look promising. I believe that maintaining a high level of NEAT is very much an authentic pattern of human behaviour that underpins optimal health. To support such a view, we need not look further than the Amish. The Amish are a christian group based in the states of Ohio, Pennsylvania, and Indiana and frozen in the 19th century. Amish communities consider working hard to be godly, and as a result they consider modern technology undesirable as it reduces the need for hard work. There is no internet, no phones, no cars, and they have even rejected machines such as automatic floor cleaners for the large barns as they liberate too much free time. Therefore, one may reach the conclusion that levels of NEAT are never lacking in Amish communities, and the data supports such a claim. On average, non-Amish US adults walk 5100 steps per day; Amish adults walk more than triple that figure with 18,000 steps per day. By prioritising hard work, the Amish are also prioritising NEAT, and perhaps because of this only four percent of Amish adults are obese. In Amish communities, NEAT is high, and obesity is very low. There are several other factors at play, but there's no doubt that the abundance of physical activity is helping to keep them lean.

Introducing a little NEAT into the mix is easy. For those struggling with obesity, it could make all the difference, as researchers from the Mayo Clinic demonstrated. They took twenty volunteers, ten lean and ten obese, and observed their activity over ten days with the instructions not to do anything that was not part of their daily routine. Throughout the ten-day period, the obese volunteers spent longer periods of time sitting down compared to the lean volunteers. The researchers concluded that if the obese volunteers emulated the daily activity of the lean volunteers, they could increase their daily energy expenditure by 350 calories. Over time, this elevated calorie burn could make a world of difference.

If we regard increasing physical activity as one of the main strategies for combating the obesity crisis, why has no one mentioned *fasting*? Because they have not evolved from the out-dated way of thinking. What we must do is take a step outside the box and gain a fresh perspective. As we discussed before, fasting is an excellent way to increase NEAT, because of how fasting stimulates orexin, the hormone responsible for wakefulness. Scientists regard orexin as a pivotal player in increasing NEAT and preventing obesity. When researchers remove orexin from mice, it decreases movement and leads to obesity. But if they *increase* orexin, it raises NEAT and improves several health markers.

Increasing NEAT with fasting offers a clear pathway to make progress for those struggling with obesity. Once you win a small battle, it becomes easier to win the next one, and this can be a powerful catalyst to break out of the vicious cycle of obesity.

GENETIC CRAVINGS, BRAIN SCANS, AND EMOTIONAL EATING

The more you eat, the less flavor;
the less you eat, the more flavor.

- CHINESE PROVERB

A fundamental element of the obesity crisis is how our physiology reacts with the vast array of highly processed and hyper-palatable foods that are now available in abundance.

The desire for calorie-dense foods is a hard-wired survival adaptation.

Think about it.

Our hunter-gatherer ancestors would not venture out and put their lives on the line to find low-calorie options. Oh no. They had to get the most bang for their buck, because they could never guarantee the next meal. Hence why Mother Nature has programmed our genetic instructions to search out and consume calorie-dense foods. The problem is, our genetics have not kept pace with our cultural evolution. Mother Nature designed humans to seek calorie-dense foods, and now we live in a world in which they surround us. Being surrounded by all this food is not an authentic pattern of human behaviour, and we can see the damage it is causing. You cannot take a dog into the butchers and expect them not to eat the meat. With humans, it's a similar situation regarding our instincts and this modern world. The way we live today is not compatible with our genetic conditioning, and an important factor in this is the brain.

Scientists suggest that insulin resistance, a common characteristic of obesity, influences how an individual behaves around food by altering motivation-reward pathways in the brain. To shed light on how obesity and insulin resistance interact with the brain, let's dive into a study from the Yale University School of Medicine. The researchers hypothesized that obese and insulin resistant individuals would show *more* brain activity in response to stress and favourite food cues than lean individuals. They took fifty participants and split them into two conditions, lean and obese, and measured their levels of insulin resistance. To avoid generic conditions, they asked each participant their favourite foods and what they find stressful beforehand to develop personalised cues. The participants then underwent an fMRI scan during exposure to their individualised food and stress cues. Compared to the lean group, the obese participants showed increased brain activity in response to the cues, with the highest activation correlated to those with the highest levels of insulin resistance. And what is the best way to reduce insulin resistance? *Fasting*.

When we see the manner in which obesity and insulin resistance can affect brain activity around food and stress, it paves the way for a whole new avenue of understanding. I recall someone close to me who was struggling with their weight getting stressed about insignificant matters. And how they would come alive when we would prepare to sit down and dine on their favourite meal. As if they were on an ecstatic high from drugs. This shift in mood was fascinating, and I would often theorise that the brain must light up like crazy in a certain way when this person encountered their favourite food. The science shows that the various mechanisms of obesity alter brain activity, and this is another reason why we should hesitate before we pass judgement on those struggling. It's all too easy to blame obesity on a lack of willpower or dedication, but once again we can see that this kind of attitude is far too reductionist. By incorporating fasting, and reducing insulin resistance, we can make moves to get the brain back on our side and striking out of the vicious cycle.

Another factor we forget in obesity is *stress*. As we saw in the study, various alterations in brain activity can make those struggling with obesity more susceptible to stress. Not only are higher levels of stress linked to difficulty losing weight, but elevated stress can cause emotional eating and further cravings, which leads to more weight gain, more stress and more cravings. It is another manifestation of this vicious cycle. Psychological stress is an integral factor in our eating behaviour and food choices. This kind of stress triggers a release of ghrelin, the hunger hormone, and amplifies our hard-wired desire for calorie-dense foods. Psychological stress leads to comfort eating. And this is a subject where science and common sense are in total agreement: comfort food is comforting to those who are the most stressed. What are comfort foods? They are calorie dense and hyper-palatable i.e. the food that our genetics have conditioned us to seek e.g. pizza and doughnuts. Reducing psychological stress is universally beneficial, but for those struggling with obesity, getting a handle on it is a pivotal step in breaking out of the vicious cycle.

I posit that fasting is a great method of avoiding psychological stress because:

- Fasting reduces decision fatigue, and fewer decisions means less stress.

- Having to worry about what to eat every few hours generates a considerable amount of stress. Fasting deletes this.

- It is much less stressful to *abstain* from something for a certain amount of time rather than attempt to moderate it. Fasting works because it is easier to eat nothing at all, rather than allow oneself to eat a small amount of what they desire and risk setting off the cravings.

- Overall, fasting reduces the total exposure to food stimuli. If you are not eating, you will not be around food, and this decreases the likelihood of the food-induced cravings or stress.

Fasting reduces stress and increases insulin sensitivity, helping to bring cravings under control.

SUMMARY

We *must* consider fasting when discussing how to combat obesity. Perhaps one day, we will look back as a society and say:

It makes so much sense! How did we not consider fasting sooner?

Or perhaps we won't.

Either way, we need to get our act together soon. This problem will not solve itself if we continue doing what we are doing now.

Since 1975, worldwide obesity rates have tripled. In 2016, 13% of the world's adult population (11% of men and 15% of women) were obese. In the same year, 340 million children aged five to nineteen were overweight or obese. Much like with type 2 diabetes, obesity is *preventable*, yet the numbers continue to rise. It begs the question: *what on earth are we doing to ourselves?*

We must expand the conversation and explore new avenues on how to stem the prevalence of obesity. It's time to emulate authentic patterns of human behaviour and embrace fasting.

PARACELSUS AND THE MYSTERIOUS HORMONE

The art of healing comes from nature, not from the physician.
Therefore the physician must start from nature,
with an open mind.

- PARACELSUS

Philippus Aureolus Theophrastus Bombastus von Hohenheim, or Paracelsus for short, was born in Switzerland in 1493 and is widely regarded as one of the three fathers of modern medicine. Carl Jung, a renowned psychologist and also Swiss, echoed this view, writing:

We see in Paracelsus not only a pioneer in the domains of chemical medicine, but also in those of an empirical psychological healing science.

Paracelsus changed the game. And according to his work he was a bold proponent of fasting. As he wrote 500 years ago: *'fasting is the greatest remedy, the physician within'*. High praise. I wonder: to what type of ailment was he referring to exactly when he spoke of remedies? Perhaps he was talking about the anti-inflammatory properties of fasting, considering that inflammation can cause and advance many diseases.

The inflammatory response is a defence mechanism in which the immune system recognizes and removes harmful stimuli and starts the healing process.

Acute inflammation is like the swelling of a bruise and is a natural part of the healing process.

Chronic inflammation is not so obvious, however, and can build up over many months or years to cause serious health complications.

Within scientific circles, there is a growing consensus that fasting can reduce several inflammatory markers and therefore be a powerful practice for combatting various common diseases. Consultation of the animal data routinely shows the anti-inflammatory potential of fasting, but let's see if we can find any human examples.

Rheumatoid arthritis causes long-term pain, swelling and stiffness in the joints, and is one example of an auto-immune condition that stems from inflammation.

Let's step back to 1988 and consider a fascinating study from the Karolinska Institute in Stockholm, Sweden. The researchers monitored fourteen patients with rheumatoid arthritis before, during, and after a seven day fasting period. After a week, all fourteen patients reported that their arthritis pain had eased. Seven days is a long fast, and perhaps an extreme measure, but it shows us that fasting is doing *something* positive. And if we go back even further to 1880, we can detect a similar theme.

Henry Tanner was a forlorn physician who had become increasingly disillusioned with life towards the end of the 1800s. A combination of his wife leaving him and unbearable pain from his arthritis led him to decide to take his own life. During his formative years, they taught him that going without food for ten days would cause death. He thought it would be oh-so easy, but after ten days of fasting, he found that rather than being dead; he felt quite the opposite. He felt *alive*, and it had eased him from the previously constant pain of his arthritis. Tanner famously fasted for forty days in front of a live audience and regularly prescribed therapeutic fasting to his patients. As reported in the *Brooklyn Daily Eagle*, Henry Tanner declared at 83 that his health was invariably *excellent*, and he would live eight further years, passing away at 91.

Inflammation causes undesirable flare-ups of psoriasis. In 2019, an international group of scientists set out to examine if Ramadan fasting would impact psoriasis. Researchers asked subjects observing Ramadan to rate their psoriasis on the Psoriasis Area and Severity Index (PASI)* on three occasions: before, during and after the holy month. Once the study period was complete, the researchers collected all the reported scores and compared them. The graph below shows the results.

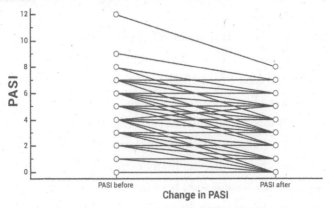

As you can see, most subjects reported that their psoriasis improved by the end of the month. There are various limitations with studies done on Ramadan, as they are not tightly controlled which allows for other factors to affect the results , but it is still an interesting finding.

While the evidence is not concrete just yet, it suggests that fasting has some anti-inflammatory potential, but I suppose the question is: *why?* From an evolutionary perspective, the anti-inflammatory properties of fasting make sense. Not having to worry about inflammation and the various complications that stem from it would have been a survival advantage for Zug and his chums during prolonged periods of food scarcity, but we may have to get a little

---

*the most widely used tool for the measurement of severity of psoriasis. PASI combines the assessment of the severity of lesions and the area affected into a single score in the range 0 (no disease) to 72 (maximal disease).

more scientific.

For starters, research has shown that ketone bodies can reduce inflammation. Considering that the body is running primarily on ketone bodies during prolonged fasting, this would help to explain why longer fasts seem to have a more potent anti-inflammatory effect. Fasting also lowers the level of c-reactive protein, which is one of the main inflammatory markers. In a study that observed subjects adhering to a 16/8 fasting protocol for eight weeks, researchers discovered that various inflammatory markers had decreased. They attributed this anti-inflammatory effect to the increase of a hormone called *adiponectin*.

You may not have heard of adiponectin before, and you may just have to repeat it a few times to get the hang of it. Ah-di-poh-neck-tin. Scientists only discovered adiponectin in the 1990s, and while it is still mysterious, it is becoming an important area of research in the realm of obesity and chronic disease. Many even suggest that adiponectin may be one of the *missing links* between obesity and the subsequent increase in risk for diabetes, heart disease, and cancer. Adiponectin is anti-inflammatory, but it may have some other tricks up its sleeve.

It would appear that getting this mysterious hormone under control could have broad implications for human health. In a scientific review that attempted to shed light on the subject, lead author Manju Chandran M.D concluded:

Although further investigations are required, adiponectin administration, as well as regulation of the pathways controlling its production, represents a promising target for managing obesity, hyperlipidemia, insulin resistance, type 2 diabetes, and vascular inflammation.

Our hard-to-pronounce friend has some powerful potential, but just *what* is adiponectin all about? In the obese, adiponectin is *low*. When we consult the data, we see that it routinely associates low levels of adiponectin with obesity. Emerging research continues to suggest that adiponectin can play an important role in the management and potential reversal of obesity and various other conditions, and the scientists are beginning to agree. But *why?* The main reason for this would be that adiponectin likes to burn fat. Stimulated adiponectin results in an elevated breakdown of fat for fuel.

This talented hormone attaches itself to another good friend of ours: leptin. When adiponectin goes up, leptin goes down. Levels of leptin are already unusually high in obese individuals, which often leads to leptin resistance. Therefore, being able to lower levels of leptin with adiponectin offers a pathway to decrease the resistance, strengthen the satisfaction signal, and break out of the vicious cycle. This would also help to explain why obesity researchers view adiponectin as such a promising area of study. In a similar vein, adiponectin is a natural insulin *sensitiser*, as it activates several pathways that operate to reduce insulin resistance. While it would appear that adiponectin attacks fat, it also protects the heart, with various studies documenting the cardiovascular protective properties of this enigmatic agent. All rather exciting, however, let's not get too carried away. At this stage, we must remind ourselves that adiponectin is still rather mysterious in the sense that we do not know a lot about it. However, with all things considered, it is interesting information to marinate on.

Miyao Matsubara, a Japanese scientist and adiponectin researcher, believes that adiponectin could be a game changer, as he concludes in one study:

Supplementation of adiponectin in insulin resistance and obesity may possibly become standard treatment for these diseases.

If we consider that fasting can stimulate adiponectin, then perhaps one day, we could consider the humble fasting as a standard treatment for 'these diseases' too. Or at the very least, as a good place to start.

FREEDOM

The constant desire for more freedom
ironically limits us in a number of ways.
Similarly, it's only by limiting ourselves - by choosing
and committing to certain things in life
- that we truly exercise our freedom.

- MARK MANSON

There are several benefits to fasting, but one of the most powerful is often one of the most overlooked: the *freedom* that comes with it.

I'm Scottish, so I had to talk about freedom.

Embracing fasting is about shedding layers that are weighing us down and becoming a more efficient version of ourselves that is unfazed by the insignificant worries of the world. It liberates us from the control of food as we no longer have to worry so much about what, when and where we will eat. Fasting is freedom from nutritional dogma and stale beliefs. It's a special freedom that empowers us to go against the grain and challenge the status quo with confidence.

When discussing the legality of certain psychedelic plants, the late Terence McKenna, a popular advocate for the responsible use of such plants, hypothesized that they were illegal because *'they open you up to the possibility that everything you know is wrong'.* Whether you agree with Terence is another debate entirely, but we *can* agree that opening ourselves up to the possibility that we have been wrong is a powerful experience that provides an opportunity for growth.

When I first heard about fasting, I was sceptical.

'*There is no way I could go twelve hours without eating,*' was a phrase I uttered during my pre-fasting days. However, I would like to think I've always had something of an open mind, so I tried it, and the experience was different from what I had expected.

When I let fasting into my life, it opened me up to the possibility that I had been wrong about many things, and I had no choice but to let my guard down and accept it. I had to accept that I was wrong, and it's been one of the best things that has ever happened to me. Realising that I was wrong and that I must ask more questions and not believe everything I'm told has been of immeasurable benefit to me in both my personal and my professional life.

You only have to prove yourself wrong once, and then the journey of discovery can move up the gears.

TIME PRESSURE, STALE CROISSANTS, AND THICKER WALLETS

Focus is the art of knowing what to ignore.
The fastest way to raise your level of performance:
Cut your number of commitments in half.

- JAMES CLEAR

Once upon a time, there was just never enough *time*.

Not so long ago, food enslaved me. And mainstream media brainwashed me into believing that I must consume breakfast in the morning. As a result, I often had to deal with the common dilemma: lose time or lose money?

I either had to wake up earlier than usual to squeeze in some kind of breakfast before work, or buy something on my way in to the office. Breakfast was always a pain in the proverbials, but since I've incorporated fasting, I don't worry about it anymore, which has not only saved me time, but it has also thickened my wallet somewhat. Have you ever stayed at a hotel and paid extra for a breakfast that left you feeling *underwhelmed?* A stale croissant and a glass of juice, perhaps? Breakfast is big business, but we rarely get any bang for our buck. More often than not, it's just a glorified dessert and a complete waste of money and time. Eating as soon as we wake up is no way to start the day. The best way to start the day is to just *start* the day and get moving, no croissant necessary. Fasting has the power to simplify life and save time.

I used to worry a lot about food. And I invested plenty of time and mental energy into deliberating over what to eat, when to eat, how to prepare it, how much I will pay and whether it was healthy. Until I discovered fasting, I never realised quite how much time food was consuming from my life. Eating is delightful, and we should celebrate it, but it need not be on the mind all throughout the day.

In a study published in *The Journal of Business Ethics*, researchers found that 'the experience of time affluence was positively related to subjective well-being'. Having a bit of time to spare and not feeling rushed can bring a significant amount of happiness. On the other hand, feeling *pressed* for time can have serious consequences regarding our health and wellbeing. One study published in the *Journal of Health and Social Behaviour* found that excessive time pressure made people more prone to anxiety and depression. Not only that, but researchers from the Australian National University ranked time pressure among the most influential social trends that contribute to the rising rates of obesity.

How many times have you heard someone blame a lack of time for their inability to take control of their nutrition? *I just don't have the time to eat well* is the familiar mantra often echoed by the time pressed individual as they seize another slice of pizza. Researchers from the University of Minnesota found that participants who experienced more perceived time pressures, such as a longer working week, found it harder to eat well. It is a struggle to eat well on the run, but *fasting* on the run is rather straightforward.

We have the power to change the situation; we just need to exercise it. Everyone complains about a lack of time, but the solution is right in front of us. Fasting can save us a great deal of time, and in doing so, help to secure our health and our happiness. Saving time makes sustainable fat loss a doddle, and it can even save lives, or at the very least make them much more enjoyable. It could well save you a bit of *cash*, too.

Let's pause and consider all the expensive items people buy just because they believe that eating at certain times is compulsory.

Buying food on the run is expensive.

Buying food in the airport, on the plane, or on board any form of transport is expensive.

Buying food *all the time* is expensive.

But it's all *nonsense*.

Embrace the freedom of fasting to reduce stress and save time and money. Invest that cash in expanding the bookshelf instead, you will need something to do with all that newfound time.

SOCIAL FREEDOM, SHEDDING LAYERS, AND BECOMING WHO YOU ARE

The object of life is not to be on the side of the majority,
but to escape finding oneself in the ranks of the insane.

- MARCUS AURELIUS

You can read a lot of nonsense on the Internet.

I recall scrolling through Instagram and coming across quite an aggressive post from a self-proclaimed health and fitness *expert* insisting that people should not do intermittent fasting and supplying ten reasons to support the claim. Most of these reasons were absolute *piffle*. Number seven in particular was high on the piffle scale:

Intermittent fasting ruins your life because you can't be spontaneous or social because of adherence to strict eating windows.

But the reality is quite the opposite. For starters, the fasting windows need only be as strict as you make them. As we discussed before, fasting windows are *flexible* and we can manipulate them around social commitments. Fasting gives you calorie freedom, which equates to *social* freedom. Consider the following scenario.

Mo and Dave have a party tonight. Mo fasts for most of the day, whereas Dave elects to eat at regular intervals from the moment he wakes up. At the party, Mo has the calorie freedom, because he's been fasting all day. Dave does not, because he's been *eating* all day. Mo can eat and drink more or less whatever he likes without risk of going overboard. Dave's lack of calorie freedom limits him to just one beer, making him a nervous wreck. If you are fasting for most of the day, then you will have more calories to play with than someone who has been eating throughout the whole day. For that big dinner or party, this difference could prove crucial.

No one wants to worry about what they can or can't eat or drink or stress over the menu when the festivities are in full flow. With the calorie freedom that fasting brings, it's a lot harder to overindulge, so you can be more impulsive, more present, and much more fun. Therefore, I believe that fasting is in fact a central component of social freedom because of the calorie freedom that it brings to the table.

I would also posit that fasting can enhance the holidaying experience. To help me explain why that is, I'll share with you the details of Mo's last week off. Don't worry; it doesn't get naughty.

Mo has gone to Copenhagen for the week. *Why*, you ask? Well, there's a lot of sights, the food is amazing and the Danish speak better English than most British people do. The allure of the danish pastry is strong, but does Mo *have* to eat it in the morning? Will Mo be fasting during his holiday? On his voyage to Copenhagen, Mo wants to:

a) See the sights.

b) Enjoy the food and beer

Fasting enables him to enjoy both to the maximum. Allow me to explain.

Mo rises from his slumber bright and early, ready for a day of adventures. He freshens up and reviews his itinerary for the day over a simple black coffee. Within a half hour, Mo is already out the door and getting the day started; no need to worry about breakfast. Mo spends the day seeing the sights and notching up plenty of steps. He loves walking in the fasted state. In fact, he finds that he is more energetic and perceptive while fasting, which makes it the perfect accompaniment to a busy day of sightseeing. As the evening approaches, Mo gets back to his place with plenty of time to get spruced up before dinner. Seeing as he racked up incredible amounts of NEAT with all that walking and talking, Mo now has calorie freedom to enjoy himself when he goes out. Mo plans to eat and drink to his heart's content. Considering that he saved some serious cash by sticking to water throughout the day, he even has the funds to treat the nice local girl that he met in Tivoli Gardens.

I often get asked if I fast *even* while on holiday.

My answer? *Of course.*

Something else that you may come to realise when you embrace fasting and experience the reality of it is that many people are just *repeaters*. I know I was. They repeat things they see on TV, that they read in magazines or on social media, or perhaps that someone down the pub told them. Repeat, repeat, repeat. As if it's stone cold fact. But they never dig deeper to discover the truth.

Eat six meals a day to lose weight: **repeat.**

Breakfast is the most important meal of the day: **repeat.**

You must eat before exercise for energy: **repeat.**

Fasting is unhealthy and unnatural: **repeat.**

It's nonsense. Most people have forgotten to look at it with a critical eye. They are just *repeating*.

Repeating is dangerous because it locks a person into being swayed by mainstream media and popular opinion, and they neglect to use their own mind. When you embrace fasting, you can break free from this pattern of repeating. Embracing fasting leads you to a path of enquiry that requires questioning everything, as opposed to blind belief. In the age of *fake news*, this could be invaluable.

Life is like a game of Tetris; the more you try to fit in, the more likely you are to disappear. Fasting forces you to ask more questions, and to not believe something just become someone says it. Fasting is Mother Nature's way of *waking us up*. It may also be a way to connect with ourselves on a much deeper level.

As we make our way through life, we pick up several layers of negativity that weigh us down and prevent us from aiming high. Fasting breaks down many preconceived notions and self-imposed limitations. In doing so, it allows us to shed these various doubts, dependencies and concocted limitations from our shoulders and move closer to self-actualisation. For example, let's say that you thought fasting was *impossible*. However, after a little experimentation, you find that you can fast with ease. You can do something that you said you could not, so it begs the question: what other limitations have you imposed on yourself?

'I can't do this.'

'I can't do that.'

'It will never work.'

'It's not worth it.'

'I don't like that.'

'I'm too young.'

'I'm too old.'

'It's too late.'

'I can't change.'

'It's just the person I am.'

'I'll never be who I want to be.'

Nonsense.

It's all an illusion.

You can do anything, and you can be whoever you want to be.

Even reaching the moon is possible. Unlikely yes, but possible. If you set small achievable goals and stay consistent over the long-term, then you can do anything. Building self-confidence is just about doing what you thought you couldn't do, over and over again. Until you understand that your mind creates limits that don't exist in reality.

It's time to become the best version of yourself.

It's time to *change the game*.

SUMMARY

Fasting is freedom.

People often overlook this aspect of fasting as they are too concerned about the specifics of fat loss. But it is perhaps the greatest benefit that fasting can offer. It's easy to fall into the trap of thinking we can only improve life through addition. We forget that *subtraction* offers happiness too. There are many voices in this world that encourage us to add. But they do so because it benefits them, not us. Mainstream media, corporations, social media influencers: they are all at it to ensure that their profit margins stay healthy. The secret, however, could be to focus on *subtraction*. It's much cheaper, too.

Fasting is *simple*.

And life is beautiful when we keep it simple.

THE GOODLIFE PHILOSOPHY

Simple can be harder than complex:
You have to work hard to get your thinking clean to make it simple.
But it's worth it in the end because once you get there,
you can move mountains.

- STEVE JOBS

There will never be one approach that suits everyone. However, there are some basic guidelines that I feel can be universally empowering.

- Energy balance is ultimately the deciding factor in weight loss or gain. We need not live by it religiously, but it reinforces the fact that there is no need to demonise certain foods or adhere to extreme restrictions.

- Use the fasting schedule as a tool to *enhance* your enjoyment of day-to-day life, rather than take away from it. Remember, flexibility is key.

- Don't take the pursuit of a healthy lifestyle or adherence of fasting windows to an extreme. This type of obsessive behaviour is known as *orthorexia*. It's a lot more common than you may think, and it can be damaging psychologically. Food should be enjoyed and meals shared with family and friends. If your 'healthy' lifestyle prevents you from doing this, then perhaps it's not so healthy after all.

- Regarding what is acceptable to drink during a fast or whether something will break it, just keep it as simple as possible. One of the most beautiful things about fasting is how much it can simplify life, so don't deny yourself this benefit by getting caught up in complications.

- Make adjustments in your daily life to prioritise NEAT.

- Start some form of resistance training. Lifting weights is healthy *and* therapeutic.

- Prioritise protein. (unless following a diet that has limitations on intake, e.g. the ketogenic diet)

- Experiment with prolonged fasting by all means, but remember that you do not *have* to do it to see results. The results will come from long-term lifestyle changes. While there may be some interesting health benefits, particularly in the realm of autophagy, there is still a lot we don't know about it. However, for all the potential benefits, it's important to remember that prolonged fasting is still a stressor, so we should not do it too often.

Part Seven

FEED THE POSITIVE, STARVE THE NEGATIVE

FEED THE POSITIVE, STARVE THE NEGATIVE

Birds born in a cage think flying is an illness.

- ALEJANDRO JODOROWSKY

Dear fellow faster,

Following your decision to implement some kind of fasting, I am in no doubt that you have received a fair share of criticism during the journey.

Let me be clear. There is always a place for constructive criticism and discussion, and we should always welcome reasonable debate.

We are all open-minded, peaceful people here.

However, many of the criticisms levelled at fasting are far from reasonable. Critics can become aggressive in their quest to inform us of how wrong and stupid they think we are, and this behaviour is not on.

It's just not *cricket*, is it?

I have chosen some of the most frequent criticisms I have received in my time alongside some common questions that people often have when they experiment with fasting, and constructed model answers for each of them. Please store them in the mental bank and recite them whenever the need arises to extinguish any negativity.

Let the respectful rebuttals begin.

Warm regards,

Scott

'I could never do that'

I'm afraid to say you are mistaken with this pessimistic assessment. Let me tell you why that is.

Not only can you fast, but you can do so much more. Fasting is easy, and once you realise this, life becomes much smoother.

Honestly.

Physically, fasting is a doddle. Although it's strange to deal with the hunger waves at first, these subside within a few weeks and it becomes a very natural process. Mentally, I concede it can be a little more challenging, and there are two reasons for this.

The first is all the tempting distractions in the modern world. The second is that societal norms have conditioned us to eat whenever we have the slightest urge to do so. It's difficult to overcome these obstacles, and it requires discipline, but it only gets easier with time, and when you free yourself from these restrictions, the knock-on effect is huge.

Adhering to intermittent fasting and using it as a foundation for a sustainable healthy lifestyle requires conquering a mental battlefield rigged with doubts and negativity. It can be tough at first, and many people decide not to continue with it, but with time, it becomes easy to the point of being almost *effortless*. Once you claim this victory, it will equip you to deal with any negativity in all the other areas of life.

Many people think fasting is too hard and something they cannot do. But they *can* do it. And once they experience this for themselves, they will realise that they can do so much more than they give themselves credit for.

Once you break one boundary, it becomes much easier to break another.

'I tried intermittent fasting for a week and I didn't see any results/ I didn't like it'

When you keep searching for ways to change your situation
for the better, you stand a chance of finding them.
When you stop searching, assuming they can't be found,
you guarantee they won.

- ANGELA DUCKWORTH

Whenever someone says this to me, I always have to ask:

What were you expecting?

Intermittent fasting is all about creating a healthy *lifestyle*. It is *not* a quick-fix, although that seems to be what everyone is looking for these days.

If someone judges intermittent fasting after just one week, then it is not a surprise that it doesn't score well. One week is not a realistic timeframe. You *can* achieve amazing things in a week. However, creating a healthy lifestyle is not one of them. We should incorporate fasting as part of a lifestyle, because if we are comfortable maintaining it for life, then does it matter whether we see results within a week?

We have plenty of time.

You *can* lose a lot of weight in one week. You could eat nothing but celery, or even just fast for a whole week, but would that be sustainable? Absolutely not. When it's over, you go back to your original ways, and this is where most people get frustrated.

We *have* to think of the big picture.

The first week I started going to the gym I was aching so much I couldn't even get out of bed. But if I was to judge lifting weights from just that week, then I would never have continued.

Likewise, I wasn't able to pack on 10 lbs on muscle mass within the first week, nor did I expect to. Making progress, and attaining lasting results, takes *time*.

And then, we have to discuss why someone might not like intermittent fasting during the first week. It is important to remember that the vast majority of people on earth have become accustomed to eating frequently throughout the day. When we take the body out of this pattern of behaviour and throw it into something new, it will not like it. Similar to being thrown into a freezing cold lake after sitting in a sauna. Implementing fasting can be a bit of a shock to the system, and it may be a rocky road to begin with. The body now has to become accustomed to relying on another fuel source for sustained periods of time, which is something it may never have had to do before. Because of this, it can kick and scream, but it will come round with a large smile and thank you for the experience in due time.

Trust me.

Don't give intermittent fasting a week, give it *at least* a month.

At that point however, you may never look back.

'I love eating too much to do intermittent fasting'

In anything, there has to be that moment of fasting, really, in order to enjoy the feast.

- STEPHEN HOUGH

I hear this one often.

Many people often associate intermittent fasting with eating drastically less, but this is almost never the case, or at least it shouldn't be, assuming that we implement it correctly.

I love eating, probably more than anyone I know. With fasting in my life, I enjoy food much more. Rather than disappointing myself regularly with small meals or having to worry about whether everything is healthy, I can instead look forward to big, satisfying feasts. Also, given that meal time now becomes something of a special occasion, I am a lot more *present* when I eat. I'm grateful for the experience, and I enjoy every moment.

If someone *loves* to eat, will they prefer big meals comprising foods that make their heart sing, or frequent small meals that barely make a dent in their appetite? I know which one I prefer.

Fasting allows us to enjoy our food without the guilt and worry. Ironically, it could be the perfect match for someone who loves to eat.

'I think about food too much to do intermittent fasting'

The philosophy of fasting calls upon us to know ourselves,
to master ourselves, and to discipline ourselves the better to free
ourselves.
To fast is to identify our dependencies, and free ourselves from them.

- TARIQ RAMADAN

An engaging discussion took place with a few people down at the gym the other day. We were debating the intricacies of various nutritional approaches when Frank said something that piqued my enthusiasm. He had tried intermittent fasting for a week but had to stop because he just could not stop thinking about food.

Mate, it was crazy, not one minute passed during the fasting period where I didn't think about food.

Everyone agreed and labelled fasting as just another fad, but before we could return to discussing the best way to season broccoli, I tossed a spanner into the works.

Hold on, Frank, isn't that a good reason to continue fasting?

Frank looked at me as if I had just left the weights scattered around the gym floor. But I couldn't help myself. I had to say it. Being enslaved by food is not a natural way to live.

I remember when eating was always on my mind. It wasn't just thinking about what I'd like to eat, but also planning all of those meals and snacks. And the negative side: the worry and guilt that creeps in.

When will I eat next?

Will it be a healthy choice?

How much should I eat?

Will I regret this later?

All that nonsense. I'm sure you can relate. Life is just too short to invest time worrying about such frivolous matters. All the fear-mongering brainwashed me. I cannot accept that Mother Nature designed us to be eating or thinking about food all the time. In fact, I reject this notion.

Food is amazing. The act of eating brings us together, and we should always celebrate it. Research has shown that eating in good company raises levels of oxytocin, the hormone responsible for trust and bonding, in chimpanzees. Don't forget, we share about 95% of our DNA with chimpanzees, and they have elaborate social structures that loosely resemble our own.

I love eating, but I refuse to let it *enslave* me. I've already spent far too much of my life worrying about food. It's time to take back control.

When I first started fasting, I was thinking about food a lot. Sometimes I'd get nervous watching the clock, or I would fantasise about food. This was not because of hunger or a nutritional deficiency, but conditioned behaviour. I was outside the parameters of my comfort zone and doing something foreign, so there was always going to be a few bumps in the road. Fasting has been an astute teacher and made me realise how much food dictated my daily life, but it also liberated me from that cycle. It did, however, take a little longer than a week to get over the food thoughts, but I'm glad I stuck with it. In fact, it's the best choice I ever made. Funnily enough, no one seems to bother me at the gym anymore.

Embracing fasting and liberating ourselves from the constant thought of food is an empowering experience.

Take back control of your mental bandwidth.

'But breakfast is the most important meal of the day!'

Deconstruct the word breakfast.

What do you get? Break-fast.

Break-the-fast.

Breakfast is the meal that one eats to signal the end of their fasting period. For most people, this is the end of the natural fasting period of sleep, hence why they eat it in the morning when we wake up.

I suppose that breakfast *is* a very important meal. How we break the fast is important and we should take it seriously. What I disagree with, however, is the notion that eating first thing in the morning, or as soon as we wake up, is necessary. Allow me to explain why that is.

Are you aware who coined the phrase *breakfast is the most important meal of the day*? It was, in fact, a medical doctor who went by the name John Harvey **Kellogg**. Coincidence? *I think not.*

1895 was a year of firsts.

Tchaikovsky's now world-famous ballet *swan lake* premiered in a St. Petersburg theatre. Caroline Willard Baldwin was the first female to receive a PhD in science. It was also the first time that a company would produce a processed food product on a massive scale.

In 1895, Dr. Kellogg launched Cornflakes. When he observed how much grain the farmers were discarding as waste from their average crop yield, Dr. Kellogg seized the opportunity to cash in. He was certain that he could use these leftover grains for something, so he purchased the lot and re-packaged them as a meal in a box. The grains were so devoid of nutritional value that they would spray them with artificial nutrients to fortify them. Dr. Kellogg had developed a product with a *huge* profit margin, but he now had to figure out how to sell something so banal and tasteless. He wanted to market it as an anti-masturbatory food, as he believed that Corn Flakes would stop men from masturbating. Oddly enough, this idea did not make the final cut. Luckily for him, there were two factors benefiting his cause.

The first was that in those days, they did not consider sugar unhealthy like we do now. In fact, it was quite the opposite situation, with sugar often being touted as a *champion* of health. This meant he could recommend adding copious amounts of sugar to Corn Flakes, which would help disguise their complete lack of flavor.

Second, it was much easier to pull the wool over people's eyes one hundred years ago. Nowadays, you can learn another language on YouTube, but back then there was no Internet, and it was a lot harder to gain information. And so, Dr. Kellogg set in motion one of the biggest marketing campaigns in history. He invented the mantra *breakfast is the most important meal of the day* to sell cereals and nothing more. It was *not* part of an honest public health initiative. They handed out pamphlets with pro-breakfast propaganda and radio adverts reminded everyone to eat their breakfast or risk the consequences. The Kellogg's propaganda machine made skipping breakfast socially unacceptable, and this attitude is still prevalent in society today. Have you ever stopped to think about just how *cheap* it is to manufacture cereal? That it's still so popular is almost as scandalous as the pricing. There is no reliable evidence to support the notion that eating cereal first thing in the morning is beneficial.

I mean, who even eats cereal anymore?

It's time to wake up. And skip breakfast.

At this stage, I must again remind you of something very important: *Just because everyone says a thing is true, does not always make it so.*

'Intermittent fasting is a fad diet'

There is nothing new, except what has been forgotten

- MARIE ANTOINETTE

This one is *easy*.

A *fad* is something that comes out of nowhere, takes the world by storm, and then fades into obscurity afterwards. However, even the staunchest critic would have to admit that fasting has been around since the dawn of time. It was part of several ancient cultures and many religions still practice it today. Fasting is not a fad. It's just that many of us have forgotten about it, that's all.

Second, fasting is not a diet. Diets are all about *what* to eat. Fasting is all about *when* to eat. And that's not to mention that, for most people, fasting is a lifestyle component. Therefore, we cannot consider intermittent fasting as a diet.

Fasting:

Not a *fad*.

Not a *diet*.

Not a *fad diet*.

'People keep telling me that intermittent fasting is unhealthy and I shouldn't do it'

Dogs bark at what they don't understand

- HERACLITUS

NOISE LEVELS

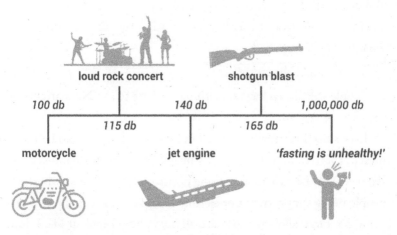

Let's talk about dealing with *negativity*.

On my 18th birthday, a man with an axe threatened me. *Really*. It was a sunny July afternoon. I was with some close friends in a pub. And I was rather intoxicated. As my friends and I stumbled out of the establishment, a big Range Rover with blacked-out windows drove past. As it did, I shouted:

John Terry!

Now why would I do such a thing? Well, we were near the training ground of Chelsea Football Club, of whom John Terry was the captain at the time. I had also seen John driving a similar car only days before. Sometimes, when you've had a few, your brain makes these kinds of connections. I'm sure you understand. I thought it was rather innocuous, but the driver of the range rover did not. Spoiler alert: it wasn't John Terry. Or his Range Rover. The car stopped in the middle of the road, and a plump man wearing sunglasses jumped out wielding an axe with a bright orange handle. He came up close to me and asked me what I had said. A mixture of fear and inebriation meant that I couldn't get my words together to formulate a coherent response. Within seconds, the angry gentleman ran back to his car and drove off. My friends and some passers-by flocked around me to ask me if I was okay. I was fine. But I was struggling to understand what had just happened.

The moral of the story?

People will *always* have something negative to say. No matter what you do.

Ever since I became interested in health and fitness and bettering myself, there has always been pushback. At first, this confused me. I'm trying my best to do something positive with my life, so why aren't people being supportive? But as time has passed, I've realised what's going on. First, allow me to share with you how I look at life. I don't mind if you laugh.

You are a cosmic being of infinite potential. And you do not have the time to concern yourself with other people projecting their dissatisfaction about their own current situation. That's what the negativity is: a *reflection*. Some people hate when you change. Because it reminds them they haven't.

And how do I know this? Because I've been there myself. In the darker moments of my life, I sometimes struggled to be happy for other people. I'm ashamed to say it, but in these moments, a small part of me didn't want my friends to be too successful. Because it reminded me how much of a loser I was.

True lions don't love the circus. And if you spend your time worrying about the reflections of other people, that is precisely what life will become: a circus. Don't worry about the unhappy reflections of other people. You've got a life to live.

We should always welcome reasonable debate. If someone brings science, logic and evidence to the table, then let's have a discussion. But all the unreasonable criticisms and petty insults? You don't have time for that. Life is just too short. Some people are going to believe what they want to believe. And it would be unwise to invest time and energy trying to convince them otherwise.

Is fasting unhealthy? No. It's not. But let me tell you what *is* unhealthy: losing sleep over what other people think.

Take it all with a pinch of salt.

Preferably of the Pink Himalayan variety.

'I've hit a plateau with my weight, what should I do?'

Just because you can measure something
doesn't mean it's the most important thing.
One pitfall of modern life
is that we often measure ourselves by that which is easy to measure.
-the number on the scale
-the ROI of the portfolio
-the number of likes on a post
It is unlikely that what can be measured
is the best way to measure a life.
You are not a number.

- JAMES CLEAR

Scale weight is a flawed metric of progress.

Let's discuss why that is.

One of the most common mistakes that people make is to judge their progress solely on the number displayed by the scale. Not only is this an incomplete method of measuring progress, it is rather frustrating too. Body weight will always fluctuate. So weighing yourself every day makes little sense. The number on the scale displays your total weight, *not* your level of body fat. Your weight can change even if your level of body fat stays exactly the same. A superior strategy is to weigh yourself less and monitor long-term trends instead. Weigh yourself once a week, but compare progress once a month. This way, you can observe the general trend over a long period, rather than getting caught up in the minor fluctuations that will ultimately prove inconsequential. It will be beneficial for your sanity too.

It's also important to measure progress with other methods. Regular photos and measurements, such as waist size, are very useful indicators of body composition and are far more informative than scale weight. Judging progress according to the number on the scale and nothing else is silly. Perhaps you have plateaued on the scale, but are still making progress. You can see visible changes to your physique, but no change on the scale. If that is the case, *who cares* about the scale weight? We humans love to categorise things numerically, but in this scenario it makes little sense. The holistic approach is the way forward.

If in doubt, remind yourself of the mission. If your goal is to lose body fat, and several metrics of progress have improved, such as how your clothes fit, then who cares about the scale? More often than not, worrying about the number on the scale is a waste of energy. Measuring our weight is one tool in a box of many. So use it accordingly.

'My friend said that fasting will cause female hair loss. Is that true?'

Sometimes success is 3% brains and 97% not getting distracted by the internet.

- SHANE PARRISH

The pain in my friend's hand was so sharp that it led them to conclude that they *must* have carpal tunnel syndrome.

They went to the doctors and had the nerves over their carpal tunnel tested. The results came back negative. There was no carpal tunnel syndrome, so the doctor referred them to a physical therapist. My friend's bad posture was causing a strain in their back, leading to a pinched nerve in the shoulder and resulting in a sharp pain in the hands. We are complex beings, and when something doesn't go to plan, we need to consider *every* possibility.

Something that I often see is people being far too hasty in attributing any problems they come across during their fasting journey to the fasting itself. It's important to take a holistic approach and look at the big picture. Make sure you consider everything. What other factors have changed in your lifestyle? Have you changed your diet? Perhaps you're not eating enough or have cut out some vital nutrients? Are you remembering to take rest days from gym? Maybe your protein intake is too low? Are you experiencing more stress than usual? Getting enough sleep? These are all important elements we must take into consideration.

Keep a log of everything that has changed. This will make it a lot easier to keep track of all the different factors and isolate the variables if something goes a bit pear-shaped. If something is worrying you, please talk to your doctor. A simple blood test can reveal a lot, and much like the carpal tunnel anecdote, it may shine a light on something that was not even a consideration.

Fasting *itself* will not cause female hair loss or negatively impact the menstrual cycle. But it is not impossible that it may create a situation, like the sudden loss of weight for example, that *can* have adverse effects.

Remember, it's all about *balance*.

'How can I get back on track after a heavy weekend?'

When making plans, think big.
when making progress, think small

- JAMES CLEAR

We have all been there.

The dust has settled from another saucy weekend and feelings of guilt are creeping in. Maybe it was one drink or one pizza too many, and now there is a burning desire to get back on track. That could mean a long fast, eating only vegetables for a week or even booking a one-way ticket to Costa Rica to start a new life painting boats. These radical measures, however, are unnecessary, and I'm here to tell you why that is.

First, it is important to understand that it takes a lot to *reverse* progress.

There is only so much damage one can do in a few days, and it will never make as much as a *dent* in the overall picture of progress.

It's just a *pause*, not a rewind, so now we press play and return to business as usual.

Second, the number on the scales can deceive following an indulgent weekend, and this causes people to panic and ask something like:

I'VE JUST PUT ON (insert amount here) LBS AFTER THE WEEKEND, SHOULD I FAST FOR (insert amount here) DAYS?

Woah.

Hold on a second.

Relax.

It is impossible that most of that weight will be body fat.

In fact, chances are that most of it *isn't*.

Increasing carbohydrate or alcohol intake (both stalwarts of the naughty weekend: think beer and pizza) come with higher fluid retention, so an increase on the scale is inevitable. But remember, it's water weight, not body fat. Likewise, if one fasts throughout the week, then taking a weekend break can also result in extra fluid retention (and therefore a little weight gain). But again, it's just *water*, not fat.

Although some people like to start the week with a prolonged fast, it is critical to ensure that one is fasting for the right reasons, not for punishment.

Whatever you do, don't panic.

It's just a *pause*.

'Can fasting increase libido?'

A dying organism is often observed to be capable of
extraordinary endurance and strength.
When any living organism is attacked,
its whole function seems to aim toward reproduction.

- JOHN STEINBECK

What a lovely question to finish on. To answer it, let's consider a few factors.

The first is fasting reduces blood pressure. Various studies show the successful use of fasting to treat hypertension, which is the medical term for dangerously high blood pressure. Lowering blood pressure increases the healthy flow of blood around the body, which is key for maintaining a healthy libido in both men and women.

The second factor requires checking in with some old friends.

Growth hormone plays an important role in sexual stimulation. In 2002, researchers from the Hannover Medical School discovered this hormone is also responsible for a different growth, finding that GH plays a key role in male erectile capability. And a deficiency can cause erectile dysfunction. Research has also linked another friend of ours, orexin, to heightened sexual arousal and desire. It would appear feeling awake and feeling *horny* go hand in hand.

Everything ties back to survival, so let's frame this matter in an evolutionary context. The most crucial aspect of survival is *reproduction*. If we consider that Mother Nature activates several survival mechanisms during periods of fasting, then encouraging reproduction by stimulating libido would be one of them.

The evidence suggests fasting activates several adaptations which work to heighten sexual desire. And when we consider it from an evolutionary perspective, the claim that fasting could stimulate libido does not seem outlandish. As for my personal experience, that is perhaps a little too vulgar to share in a book that my mother is planning to read.

Fasting is all about survival adaptations, and heightening our desire to reproduce is one of them.

Every one of us is, in the cosmic perspective, precious.
If a human disagrees with you, let him live.

In a hundred billion galaxies, you will not find another.
- CARL SAGAN

The more you judge,
the more you separate yourself.

The world just reflects your own feelings back to you.
- NAVAL RAVIKANT

CLOSING

A true teacher would never tell you what to do.
But he would give you the knowledge
with which you could decide
what would be best for you to do.

- CHRISTOPHER PIKE

So here we are.

How are you feeling?

The vast majority of books in the health and fitness sphere will provide a detailed template. They tell you exactly what to do, what to eat, how long to do it for and what you can expect to happen by the end of it all. But this book does not follow such a pattern.

I don't want to tell you exactly what to do. I just want to provide some information that may change the way you look at things and empower you to make movements towards the best version of yourself.

Thriving in the third millennium will require emulating authentic patterns of human behaviour. And I believe that fasting is a great place to start. By this stage, you may agree.

I have been documenting my journey and sharing information on social media for a few years now. I regularly host Q&A sessions and love to connect with the community.

If learning more about me or my work interests you, or you would like to interact with me, you can find me on Instagram and YouTube with the username **goodlifetheory**, or on Quora under my name **Scott Murray**.

You can also have a look at my website www.goodlifetheory.com and sign up for my newsletter.

Alternatively, if you want my direct attention, you can get in touch with me via email: scott@goodlifetheory.com

Thank you for reading.

It's been a pleasure, and I look forward to connecting with you.

If you liked the book and have a few seconds spare, please leave a nice review. I would really appreciate it.

As always, much love.

Scott.

REFERENCES

Part One
Destructive Dieting

Nagasawa M et al. Oxytocin-gaze positive loop and the coevolution of human-dog bonds. *Science*. 17 Apr 2015: 333-336

Wing RR, Hill JO. Successful weight loss maintenance. *Annu Rev Nutr*. 2001;21:323-41.

Hill JO, Wyatt HR, Peters JC. Energy balance and obesity. *Circulation*. 2012;126(1):126–132.

Berns GS et al. Neurobiological correlates of social conformity and independence during mental rotation. *Biol Psychiatry*. 2005 Aug 1;58(3):245-53.

Reed GW, Hill JO. Measuring the thermic effect of food. *Am J Clin Nutr*. 1996 Feb;63(2):164-9.

Bellisle F, McDevitt R, Prentice AM. Meal frequency and energy balance. *Br J Nutr*. 1997 Apr;77 Suppl 1:S57-70.

Anton SD, Moehl K, Donahoo WT, et al. Flipping the Metabolic Switch: Understanding and Applying the Health Benefits of Fasting. *Obesity (Silver Spring)*. 2018;26(2):254–268.

Michalsen A, Li C. Fasting therapy for treating and preventing disease - current state of evidence. *Forsch Komplementmed*. 2013;20(6):444-53.

Gill S, Panda S. A smartphone app reveals erratic diurnal eating patterns in humans that can be modulated for health benefits. *Cell Metabolism*. 2015 November 3; 22(5): 789–798.

Gabel K, Hoddy KK, Haggerty N, et al. Effects of 8-hour time restricted feeding on body weight and metabolic disease risk factors in obese adults: A pilot study. *Nutr Healthy Aging*. 2018;4(4):345–353.

Part Two
Fasting for Fat Loss

SECTION ONE

Shenkin A. Micronutrients in health and disease. *Postgrad Med J.* 2006;82(971):559–567.

Carreiro AL, Dhillon J, Gordon S, et al. The Macronutrients, Appetite, and Energy Intake. *Annu Rev Nutr.* 2016;36:73–103.

NIH, National Institute of General Medical Sciences (NIGMS). The biology of fats in the body. *ScienceDaily.* 23 April 2013.

Wu G. Functional amino acids in nutrition and health. *Amino Acids.* 2013 Sep;45(3):407-11.

Dimitriadis G et al. Insulin effects in muscle and adipose tissue. *Diabetes research and clinical practice.* 2011 Aug;93 Suppl 1:S52-9.

Berg JM, Tymoczko JL, Stryer L. *Biochemistry.* 5th edition. New York: W H Freeman; 2002. Chapter 21, Glycogen Metabolism. Available from: https://www.ncbi.nlm.nih.gov/books/NBK21190/

Ameer F et al. De novo lipogenesis in health and disease. *Metabolism.* 2014; 63 (7): 895-902.

Chakrabarti P, Kim JY, Singh M, et al. Insulin inhibits lipolysis in adipocytes via the evolutionarily conserved mTORC1-Egr1-ATGL-mediated pathway. *Mol Cell Biol.* 2013;33(18):3659–3666.

Ward, Colin. Ketone body metabolism [internet]. 2015 Nov 18; Diapedia 51040851169 rev. no. 29. Available from: https://doi.org/10.14496/dia.51040851169.29

Goodpaster BH, Sparks LM. Metabolic Flexibility in Health and Disease. *Cell Metab.* 2017 May 2;25(5):1027-1036.

Thyfault JP, Rector RS, Noland RC. Metabolic inflexibility in skeletal muscle: a prelude to the cardiometabolic syndrome? *Journal of the Cardiometabolic Syndrome.* 2006 Summer;1(3):184-9.

Vieira AF et al. Effects of aerobic exercise performed in fasted v. fed state on fat and carbohydrate metabolism in adults: a systematic review and meta-analysis. *The British Journal of Nutrition*. 2016 Oct;116(7):1153-1164.

Achten J, Jeukendrup AE. Optimizing fat oxidation through exercise and diet. *Nutrition*. 2004 Jul-Aug;20(7-8):716-27.

Van Proeyen K et al. Beneficial metabolic adaptations due to endurance exercise training in the fasted state. *Journal of Applied Physiology*. 2011 Jan;110(1):236-45.

Astrup A. The relevance of increased fat oxidation for body-weight management: metabolic inflexibility in the predisposition to weight gain. *Obesity Reviews*. 2011 Oct;12(10):859-65.

Weyer C et al. Energy Expenditure, Fat Oxidation, and Body Weight Regulation: A Study of Metabolic Adaptation to Long- Term Weight Change. *Journal of Clinical Endocrinology & Metabolism*. 2000 Mar;85(3): 1087-1094.

Hoffman D et al. Why are nutritionally stunted children at increased risk of obesity? Studies of metabolic rate and fat oxidation in shantytown children from São Paulo, Brazil. *American Journal of Clinical Nutrition*. September 200;72(3); 702-707.

Jackman MR et al. Weight regain after sustained weight reduction is accompanied by suppressed oxidation of dietary fat and adipocyte hyperplasia. *American Journal of Physiology*. 2008 Apr;294(4): R1117-29.

Filozof CM et al. Low plasma leptin concentration and low rates of fat oxidation in weight-stable post-obese subjects. *Obesity Research*. 2000 May;8(3):205-10.

SECTION TWO

Klok MD, Jakobsdottir S, Drent ML. The role of leptin and ghrelin in the regulation of food intake and body weight in humans: a review.

Obesity Reviews. 2007 Jan;8(1):21-34.

Al Maskari MY, Alnaqdy AA. Correlation between Serum Leptin Levels, Body Mass Index and Obesity in Omanis. *Sultan Qaboos Univ Med J.* 2006 Dec;6(2):27-31.

Zhou Y, Rui L. Leptin signaling and leptin resistance. *Front Med.* 2013 Jun;7(2):207-22.

Boden G et al. Effect of fasting on serum leptin in normal human subjects. *J Clin Endocrinol Metab.* 1996 Sep;81(9):3419-23.

Johnstone AM et al. Effect of an acute fast on energy compensation and feeding behaviour in lean men and women. *Int J Obes Relat Metab Disord.* 2002 Dec;26(12):1623-8.

Verdich C et al. Leptin levels are associated with fat oxidation and dietary-induced weight loss in obesity. *Obesity Research.* 2001 Aug;9(8):452-61.

Müller TD et al. Ghrelin. *Mol Metab.* 2015 Mar 21;4(6):437-60.

Cummings D et al. Plasma Ghrelin Levels after Diet-Induced Weight Loss or Gastric Bypass Surgery. *N Engl J Med.* 2002; 346:1623-1630.

Rossow LM et al. Natural bodybuilding competition preparation and recovery: a 12-month case study. *Int J Sports Physiol Perform.* 2013 Sep;8(5):582-92.

Taheri S et al. Short sleep duration is associated with reduced leptin, elevated ghrelin, and increased body mass index. *PLoS Med.* 2004 Dec;1(3):e62.

Natalucci G et al. Spontaneous 24-h ghrelin secretion pattern in fasting subjects: maintenance of a meal-related pattern. *European Journal of Endocrinology.* June 2005 152(6):845-50.

Scheer FA, Morris CJ, Shea SA. The internal circadian clock increases hunger and appetite in the evening independent of food intake and other behaviors. *Obesity (Silver Spring).* 2013 Mar;21(3):421-3.

Qian J et al. Ghrelin is impacted by the endogenous circadian system and by circadian misalignment in humans. *Int J Obes (Lond).* 2019;43(8):1644–1649.

SECTION THREE

Mansoubi M, Pearson N, Clemes SA, et al. Energy expenditure during common sitting and standing tasks: examining the 1.5 MET definition of sedentary behaviour. *BMC Public Health.* 2015;15:516.

Levine JA. Non-exercise activity thermogenesis (NEAT). *Best Pract Res Clin Endocrinol Metab.* 2002 Dec;16(4):679-702.

von Loeffelholz C, Birkenfeld A. The Role of Non-exercise Activity Thermogenesis in Human Obesity. In: Feingold KR, Anawalt B, Boyce A, et al., editors. MDText.com, Inc.; 2000-. Available from: https://www.ncbi.nlm.nih.gov/books/NBK279077/

Levine JA, Eberhardt NL, Jensen MD. Role of nonexercise activity thermogenesis in resistance to fat gain in humans. *Science.* 1999 Jan 8;283(5399):212-4.

Levine JA. Nonexercise activity thermogenesis--liberating the life-force. *J Intern Med.* 2007 Sep;262(3):273-87.

Mak KK et al. Prevalence of exercise and non-exercise physical activity in Chinese adolescents. *Int J Behav Nutr Phys Act.* 2011 Jan 20;8:3.

Ebrahim IO et al. The hypocretin/orexin system. *J R Soc Med.* 2002 May;95(5):227-30.

Mahler SV et al. Motivational activation: a unifying hypothesis of orexin/hypocretin function. *Nat Neurosci.* 2014;17(10):1298–1303.

Butterick TA et al. Orexin: pathways to obesity resistance? *Rev Endocr Metab Disord.* 2013 Dec;14(4):357-64.

Ferry B, Duchamp-Viret P. The orexin component of fasting triggers memory processes underlying conditioned food selection in the rat.

Learn Mem. 2014;21(4):185–189.

Gonzalez JA et al. Inhibitory Interplay between Orexin Neurons and Eating. *Current Biology.* 2016 Sept;26:2486–2491.

Yamanaka A et al. Hypothalamic Orexin Neurons Regulate Arousal According to Energy Balance in Mice. *Neuron.* 2003 June; 38(5);701-713.

Diano S et al. Fasting activates the nonhuman primate hypocretin (orexin) system and its postsynaptic targets. *Endocrinology.* 2003 Sept;144(9):3774-8.

Almeneessier AS et al. The effects of diurnal intermittent fasting on the wake-promoting neurotransmitter orexin-A. *Ann Thorac Med.* 2018 Jan-Mar;13(1):48-54.

SECTION FOUR

Beccuti G, Pannain S. Sleep and obesity. *Curr Opin Clin Nutr Metab Care.* 2011 Jul;14(4):402-12.

Thomson CA et al. Relationship between sleep quality and quantity and weight loss in women participating in a weight-loss intervention trial. *Obesity (Silver Spring).* 2012 Jul;20(7):1419-25

Chaput JP, Tremblay A. Sleeping habits predict the magnitude of fat loss in adults exposed to moderate caloric restriction. *Obes Facts.* 2012;5(4):561-6.

Sawamoto R et al. Higher sleep fragmentation predicts a lower magnitude of weight loss in overweight and obese women participating in a weight-loss intervention. *Nutr Diabetes.* 2014 Oct 27;4(10):e144.

St-Onge MP, Shechter A. Sleep disturbances, body fat distribution, food intake and/or energy expenditure: pathophysiological aspects. *Horm Mol Biol Clin Investig.* 2014 Jan;17(1):29-37.

Morselli L et al. Role of sleep duration in the regulation of glucose metabolism and appetite. *Best Pract Res Clin Endocrinol Metab.* 2010 Oct;24(5):687-702.

Schmid SM at al. A single night of sleep deprivation increases ghrelin levels and feelings of hunger in normal-weight healthy men. *J Sleep Res.* 2008 Sep;17(3):331-4.

Benedict C et al. Acute sleep deprivation reduces energy expenditure in healthy men. *Am J Clin Nutr.* 2011 Jun;93(6):1229-36.

Pilcher JJ et al. Interactions between sleep habits and self-control. *Front Hum Neurosci.* 2015 May 11;9:284.

Greer SM, Goldstein AN, Walker MP. The impact of sleep deprivation on food desire in the human brain. *Nat Commun.* 2013;4:2259.

Rodgers CD et al. Sleep deprivation: effects on work capacity, self-paced walking, contractile properties and perceived exertion. *Sleep.* 1995 Jan;18(1):30-8.

Engle-Friedman M. The effects of sleep loss on capacity and effort. *Sleep Sci.* 2014 Dec;7(4):213-24.

Engle-Friedman M, Riela S. Self-Imposed Sleep Loss, Sleepiness, Effort and Performance. *Sleep and Hypnosis.* 2004;6(4):155-162

Medic G, Wille M, Hemels ME. Short- and long-term health consequences of sleep disruption. *Nat Sci Sleep.* 2017 May 19;9:151-161.

Washington University School of Medicine. Sleep deprivation accelerates Alzheimer's brain damage. ScienceDaily, 24 January 2019.

Cappuccio FP et al. Sleep duration and all-cause mortality: a systematic review and meta-analysis of prospective studies. *Sleep.* 2010 May 1;33(5):585-92.

Amin A et al. The central effects of thyroid hormones on appetite. *J Thyroid Res.* 2011:306510.

Fujiwara Y et al. Association between dinner-to-bed time and gastro-esophageal reflux disease. *Am J Gastroenterol.* 2005Dec;100(12):2633-6.

Lemoine P et al. Prolonged-release melatonin improves sleep quality and morning alertness in insomnia patients aged 55 years and older and has no withdrawal effects. *J Sleep Res.* 2007 Dec;16(4):372-80.

Clarke TC et al. Trends in the use of complementary health approaches among adults: United States, 2002–2012. National health statistics reports; no 79. Hyattsville, MD: National Center for Health Statistics. 2015

Peschke E, Bähr I, Mühlbauer E. Melatonin and Pancreatic Islets: Interrelationships between Melatonin, Insulin and Glucagon. *Int. J. Mol. Sci.* 2013, 14, 6981-7015.

Kline CE et al. Poor Sleep Quality is Associated with Insulin Resistance in Postmenopausal Women With and Without Metabolic Syndrome. *Metabolic Syndrome and Related Disorders.* 2018 May;16(4):183-189.

Mesarwi O et al. Sleep disorders and the development of insulin resistance and obesity. *Endocrinol Metab Clin North Am.* 2013;42(3):617–634.

Michalsen A et al. Effects of short-term modified fasting on sleep patterns and daytime vigilance in non-obese subjects: results of a pilot study. *Ann Nutr Metab.* 2003;47(5):194-200.

Sakamoto N et al. Bedtime and Sleep Duration in Relation to Depressive Symptoms among Japanese Workers. *J Occup Health.* 2013; 55: 479–486.

Fuller C et al. Bedtime Use of Technology and Associated Sleep Problems in Children. *Glob Pediatr Health.* 2017 Oct 27;4:2333794X17736972.

Orzech KM et al. Digital media use in the 2 h before bedtime is associated with sleep variables in university students. *Comput Human Behav.* 2016 Feb;55(A):43-50.

Hallegraeff JM et al. Stretching before sleep reduces the frequency and severity of nocturnal leg cramps in older adults: a randomised trial. *J Physiother.* 2012;58(1):17-22.

Bavishi A, Slade MD, Levy BR. A chapter a day: Association of book reading with longevity. *Soc Sci Med.* 2016 Sep;164:44-48.

Kang JH, Chen SC. Effects of an irregular bedtime schedule on sleep quality, daytime sleepiness, and fatigue among university students in Taiwan. *BMC Public Health.* 2009 Jul 19;9:248.

SECTION FIVE

Fond G et al. Fasting in mood disorders: neurobiology and effectiveness. A review of the literature. *Psychiatry Res.* 2013 Oct 30;209(3):253-8.

Albert PR et al. Serotonin-prefrontal cortical circuitry in anxiety and depression phenotypes: pivotal role of pre- and post-synaptic 5-HT1A receptor expression. *Front Behav Neurosci.* 2014;8:199.

Mishra A, Mishra H. We are What We Consume: The Influence of Food Consumption on Impulsive Choice (November 1, 2009). Journal of Marketing Research, Forthcoming. Available at SSRN: https://ssrn.com/abstract=1498082

Shawky S et al. Effect of Intermittent Fasting on Brain Neurotransmitters, Neutrophils Phagocytic Activity, and Histopathological Finding in Some Organs in Rats. *International Journal of Research Studies in Biosciences(IJRSB).* 3. 38-45.

Bastani A et al. The Effects of Fasting During Ramadan on the Concentration of Serotonin, Dopamine, Brain-Derived Neurotrophic Factor and Nerve Growth Factor. *Neurol Int.* 2017;9(2):7043.

Palmiter RD. Dopamine signaling as a neural correlate of consciousness. *Neuroscience.* 2011 Dec;198:21-220.

Cadman B. Dopamine deficiency: What you need to know. *Medical News Today.* MediLexicon, Intl., 17 Jan. 2018.

Drozak J, Bryła J. '[Dopamine: not just a neurotransmitter].' *Postepy Hig Med Dosw (Online).* 2005;59:405-20.

Salamone J, Correa M. The Mysterious Motivational Functions of Mesolimbic Dopamine. *Neuron.* 2012; 76 (3): 470.

Chan JL et al. Short-term fasting-induced autonomic activation and changes in catecholamine levels are not mediated by changes in leptin levels in healthy humans. *Clinical Endocrinology.* 2007 Jan;66(1):49-57.

Murphy P et al. The antidepressant properties of the ketogenic diet. *Biological Psychiatry.* 2004;56(12):981-983.

Yamanashi T et al. Beta-hydroxybutyrate, an endogenic NLRP3 inflammasome inhibitor, attenuates stress-induced behavioral and inflammatory responses. *Sci Rep.* 2017 Aug 9;7(1):7677.

Sievertsen H et al. Cognitive fatigue influences students' performance on standardized tests. *Proceedings of the National Academy of Sciences.* 2016 Mar;113(10)2621-2624.

Part Three
Your Fasting Lifestyle

SECTION ONE

Mariotti A. The effects of chronic stress on health: new insights into the molecular mechanisms of brain-body communication. *Future Sci OA.* 2015;1(3):FSO23.

Kouda K, Iki M. Beneficial effects of mild stress (hormetic effects): dietary restriction and health. *Journal of Physiological Anthropology.* 2010;29(4):127-32.

Hackney AC. Stress and the neuroendocrine system: the role of exercise as a stressor and modifier of stress. *Expert Rev Endocrinol Metab.* 2006;1(6):783–792.

Schneiderman N et al. Stress and health: psychological, behavioral, and biological determinants. *Annu Rev Clin Psychol.* 2005;1:607–628.

Mattson MP. Hormesis defined. *Ageing Res Rev.* 2008;7(1):1–7.

Coyle EF. Physical activity as a metabolic stressor. *The American Journal of Clinical Nutrition.* 2000 Aug;72(2 Suppl):512S-20S.

Lavie CJ et al. Exercise and the heart--the harm of too little and too much. *Current Sports Medicine Reports.* 2015 Mar-Apr;14(2):104-9.

Dalton A, Spiller S. Too Much of a Good Thing: The Benefits of Implementation Intentions Depend on the Number of Goals. 2012 Oct;39(3):600-614.

SECTION TWO

Higginson AD et al. Fatness and fitness: exposing the logic of evolutionary explanations for obesity. *Proc Biol Sci.* 2016 Jan 13;283(1822):20152443.

Jackson L. Physical appearance and gender: Sociobiological and sociocultural perspectives. SUNY Press, 1992.

Striegel-Moore RH et al. Gender difference in the prevalence of eating disorder symptoms. *Int J Eat Disord.* 2009 Jul;42(5):471-4.

Nair PM, Khawale PG. Role of therapeutic fasting in women's health: An overview. *J Midlife Health.* 2016 Apr-Jun;7(2):61-4.

Zangeneh F et al. The effect of Ramadan fasting on hypothalamic pituitary ovarian (HPO) axis in women with Polycystic Ovary syndrome. *Womens Health Bull.* 2014;1:e18962.

Badawy A, Elnashar A. Treatment options for polycystic ovary syndrome. *International Journal of Women's Health.* 2011 Feb 8;3:25-35.

Williams NI et al. Strenuous exercise with caloric restriction: effect on luteinizing hormone secretion. Medicine and Science in Sports and Exercise. 1995 Oct;27(10):1390-1398.

Goluch-Koniuszy ZS. Nutrition of women with hair loss problem during the period of menopause. *Prz Menopauzalny.* 2016 Mar;15(1):56-61.

National Research Council (US) Subcommittee on the Tenth Edition of the Recommended Dietary Allowances. Recommended Dietary Allowances: 10th Edition. Washington (DC): National Academies Press (US); 1989. 6, Protein and Amino Acids. Available from: https://www.ncbi.nlm.nih.gov/books/NBK234922/

Guo EL, Katta R. Diet and hair loss: effects of nutrient deficiency and supplement use. *Dermatol Pract Concept.* 2017;7(1):1–10.

McLaren DS. Skin in protein energy malnutrition. *Arch Dermatol.* 1987 Dec;123(12):1674-1676a.

Izadi V, Saraf-Bank S, Azadbakht L. Dietary intakes and leptin concentrations. *ARYA Atheroscler.* 2014;10(5):266–272.

Vázquez MJ et al. Roles of leptin in reproduction, pregnancy and polycystic ovary syndrome: consensus knowledge and recent developments. *Metabolism.* 2015 Jan;64(1):79-91.

Tena-Sempere M. Roles of ghrelin and leptin in the control of reproductive function. *Neuroendocrinology.* 2007;86(3):229-41.

Escalante Pulido JM, Alpizar Salazar M. Changes in insulin sensitivity, secretion and glucose effectiveness during menstrual cycle. *Arch Med Res.* 1999 Jan-Feb;30(1):19-22.

SECTION THREE

Shan B et al. Antioxidant capacity of 26 spice extracts and characterization of their phenolic constituents. *Journal of Agricultural and Food Chemistry.* 2005 Oct 5;53(20):7749-59.

Qin B et al. Cinnamon: potential role in the prevention of insulin resistance, metabolic syndrome, and type 2 diabetes. *J Diabetes Sci Technol.* 2010 May 1;4(3):685-93.

Gunawardena D et al. Anti-inflammatory activity of cinnamon (C. zeylanicum and C. cassia) extracts - identification of E-cinnamaldehyde and o-methoxy cinnamaldehyde as the most potent bioactive compounds. *Food & Function.* 2015 Mar;6(3):910-9.

Wakisaka S et al. The effects of carbonated water upon gastric and cardiac activities and fullness in healthy young women. *Journal of Nutritional Science and Vitaminology.* 2012 Jan;58(5):333-338.

SECTION FOUR

Ikeda A et al. Chewing Stimulation Reduces Appetite Ratings and Attentional Bias toward Visual Food Stimuli in Healthy-Weight Individuals. *Front Psychol.* 2018;9:99.

Survey of 3003 Americans, Nutrition Information Center, New York Hospital-Cornell Medical Center (April 14, 1998).

Ganio MS et al. Mild dehydration impairs cognitive performance and mood of men. *Br J Nutr.* 2011 Nov;106(10):1535-43.

Armstrong LE et al. Mild dehydration affects mood in healthy young women. *J Nutr.* 2012 Feb;142(2):382-8.

Popkin BM et al. Water, hydration, and health. *Nutr Rev.* 2010;68(8):439–458.

Maughan RJ. Impact of mild dehydration on wellness and on exercise performance. *Eur J Clin Nutr.* 2003 Dec;57 Suppl 2:S19-23.

Dennis EA, Dengo AL, Comber DL, et al. Water consumption increases weight loss during a hypocaloric diet intervention in middle-aged and older adults. *Obesity (Silver Spring).* 2010;18(2):300–307.

Soenen S, Westerterp-Plantenga MS. Proteins and satiety: implications for weight management. *Current Opinion in Clinical Nutrition and Metabolic Care.* 2008 Nov;11(6):747–751.

SECTION FIVE

Shimada K et al. Effects of post-absorptive and postprandial exercise on 24 h fat oxidation. *Metabolism: Clinical and Experimental.* 2013 Jun;62(6):793-800.

Aird TP et al. Effects of fasted vs fed-state exercise on performance and post-exercise metabolism: A systematic review and meta-analysis. *Scandinavian Journal of Medicine & Science in Sports.* 2018 May;28(5):1476-1493.

Askew EW. Role of fat metabolism in exercise. *Clinics in Sports Medicine.* 1984 Jul;3(3):605-21.

Goodpaster BH, Sparks LM. Metabolic Flexibility in Health and Disease. *Cell Metab.* 2017 May 2;25(5):1027-1036.

Van Proeyen K et al. Beneficial metabolic adaptations due to endurance exercise training in the fasted state. *J Appl Physiol.* 2011 Jan;110(1):236-45.

Nørrelund H et al. The protein-retaining effects of growth hormone during fasting involve inhibition of muscle-protein breakdown. *Diabetes.* 2001 Jan;50(1):96-104.

Velloso CP. Regulation of muscle mass by growth hormone and IGF-I. *Br J Pharmacol.* 2008 Jun;154(3):557-68.

Ganesan K et al. Intermittent Fasting: The Choice for a Healthier Lifestyle. *Cureus.* 2018 Jul 9;10(7):e2947.

Tinsley GM et al. Time-restricted feeding in young men performing resistance training: A randomized controlled trial. *European Journal of Sport Science.* 2017 Mar;17(2):200-207.

Moro T et al. Effects of eight weeks of time-restricted feeding (16/8) on basal metabolism, maximal strength, body composition, inflammation, and cardiovascular risk factors in resistance-trained males. *Journal of Translational Medicine.* 2016 14:290.

Garthe I et al. Effect of nutritional intervention on body composition and performance in elite athletes. *European Journal of Sport Science.* 2013;13(3):295-303.

Donnelly JE et al. Muscle hypertrophy with large-scale weight loss and resistance training. *American Journal of Clinical Nutrition.* 1993 Oct;58(4):561-5.

Witard OC et al. Protein Considerations for Optimising Skeletal Muscle Mass in Healthy Young and Older Adults. *Nutrients.* 2016 Mar 23;8(4):181.

Lorenz DS et al. Periodization: current review and suggested implementation for athletic rehabilitation. *Sports Health.* 2010 Nov;2(6):509-18.

Kraemer W et al. American College of Sports Medicine position stand. Progression models in resistance training for healthy adults. *Med Sci Sports Exerc.* 2002 Feb;34(2):364-80.

Aragon AA, Schoenfeld BJ. Nutrient timing revisited: is there a post-exercise anabolic window? J *Int Soc Sports Nutr.* 2013 Jan 29;10(1):5.

Wolfe RR. Branched-chain amino acids and muscle protein synthesis in humans: myth or reality? *J Int Soc Sports Nutr.* 2017;14:30.

Churchward-Venne TA, Burd NA, Mitchell CJ, et al. Supplementation of a suboptimal protein dose with leucine or essential amino acids: effects on myofibrillar protein synthesis at rest and following resistance exercise in men. *J Physiol.* 2012;590(11):2751–2765.

Ramezani Ahmadi A et al. The effect of glutamine supplementation on athletic performance, body composition, and immune function: A systematic review and a meta-analysis of clinical trials. *Clin Nutr.* 2019 Jun;38(3):1076-1091.

Onakpoya IJ et al. The efficacy of long-term conjugated linoleic acid (CLA) supplementation on body composition in overweight and obese individuals: a systematic review and meta-analysis of randomized clinical trials. *Eur J Nutr.* 2012 Mar;51(2):127-34.

SECTION SIX

Poti JM et al. Ultra-processed Food Intake and Obesity: What Really Matters for Health-Processing or Nutrient Content? *Curr Obes Rep.* 2017;6(4):420–431.

Hall K et al. Ultra-Processed Diets Cause Excess Calorie Intake and Weight Gain: An Inpatient Randomized Controlled Trial of Ad Libitum Food Intake. Cell Metabolism. May 16, 2019.

Institute of Medicine (US) Food and Nutrition Board. Frontiers in the Nutrition Sciences: Proceedings of a Symposium. Washington (DC): National Academies Press (US); 1989. The Genome: Nutrition and Human Variation. Available from: https://www.ncbi.nlm.nih.gov/books/NBK235284/

SECTION SEVEN

Stokes T. A et al. The Oddball Effect and Inattentional Blindness: How Unexpected Events Influence Our Perceptions Of Time. *Proceedings of the Human Factors and Ergonomics Society Annual Meeting.* 2017;61(1):1753–1757.

Part Four
Prolonged Fasting

SECTION ONE

Finnell JS et al. Is fasting safe? A chart review of adverse events during medically supervised, water-only fasting. *BMC Complement Altern Med.* 2018;18(1):67.

SECTION THREE

Salgin B et al. The effect of prolonged fasting on levels of growth hormone-binding protein and free growth hormone. *Growth Hormone and IGF Research: official journal of the Growth Hormone Research Society and the international IGF Research Society.* 2012 Apr;22(2):76-81.

Ho KY et al. Fasting enhances growth hormone secretion and amplifies the complex rhythms of growth hormone secretion in man. *J Clin Invest.* 1988 Apr;81(4):968-75.

Hartman ML et al. Pulsatile growth hormone secretion in older persons is enhanced by fasting without relationship to sleep stages. *The Journal of Clinical Endocrinology and Metabolism.* 1996 Jul;81(7):2694-701.

Hartman ML et al. Augmented growth hormone (GH) secretory burst frequency and amplitude mediate enhanced GH secretion during a two-day fast in normal men. *The Journal of Clinical Endocrinology and Metabolism.* 1992 Apr;74(4):757-65.

Clemmons DR et al. Growth hormone administration conserves lean body mass during dietary restriction in obese subjects. *The Journal of Clinical Endocrinology and Metabolism.* 1987 May;64(5):878-83.

Ottosson M et al. Effects of Cortisol and Growth Hormone on Lipolysis in Human Adipose Tissue. *The Journal of Clinical Endocrinology & Metabolism.* 2000 Feb;85(2):799-803.

Møller N, Jørgensen JO. Effects of growth hormone on glucose, lipid, and protein metabolism in human subjects. *Endocr Rev.* 2009 Apr;30(2):152-77.

Svensson JA, Bengtsson B. Clinical and experimental effects of growth hormone secretagogues on various organ systems. *Hormone Research.* 1999;51 Suppl 3:16-20.

Nyberg F, Hallberg M. Growth hormone and cognitive function. *Nature Reviews. Endocrinology.* 2013 Jun;9(6):357-65.

Nyberg F. Growth hormone in the brain: characteristics of specific brain targets for the hormone and their functional significance. *Frontiers in Neuroendocrinology.* 2000 Oct;21(4):330-48.

Olney RC. Regulation of bone mass by growth hormone. *Med Pediatr Oncol.* 2003 Sep;41(3):228-34.

Kuzma M, Payer J. '[Growth hormone deficiency, its influence on bone mineral density and risk of osteoporotic fractures].' (Original article in Slovak) *Casopis Lekaru Ceskych.* 2010;149(5):211-6.

Devesa J, Almengló C, Devesa P. Multiple Effects of Growth Hormone in the Body: Is it Really the Hormone for Growth? *Clin Med Insights Endocrinol Diabetes.* 2016 Oct 12;9:47-71.

Atamna H et al. Organ reserve, excess metabolic capacity, and aging. *Biogerontology.* 2018 Apr;19(2):171-184.

SECTION FOUR

Espelund U et al. Fasting Unmasks a Strong Inverse Association between Ghrelin and Cortisol in Serum: Studies in Obese and Normal-Weight Subjects. *The Journal of Clinical Endocrinology & Metabolism.* 2005 Feb;90(2):741-746.

Webber J, Macdonald IA. The cardiovascular, metabolic and hormonal changes accompanying acute starvation in men and women. *The British Journal of Nutrition.* 1994 Mar;71(3):437-47.

Mansell PI et al. Enhanced thermogenic response to epinephrine after 48-h starvation in humans. *The American Journal of Physiology.* 1990 Jan;258(1 Pt 2):R87-93.

Zauner C et al. Resting energy expenditure in short-term starvation is increased as a result of an increase in serum norepinephrine. *The American Journal of Clinical Nutrition.* 2000 June;71(6):1511-1515.

Nair KS et al. Leucine, glucose, and energy metabolism after 3 days of fasting in healthy human subjects. *The American Journal of Clinical Nutrition.* 1987 Oct;46(4):557-62.

Newsholm EA, Leech AR. Biochemistry for the medical sciences. Chichester, United Kingdom: John Wiley & Sons Ltd, 1983.

McCorry LK. Physiology of the autonomic nervous system. *Am J Pharm Educ.* 2007 Aug 15;71(4):78.

Kobayashi K. Role of catecholamine signaling in brain and nervous system functions: new insights from mouse molecular genetic study. *J Investig Dermatol Symp Proc.* 2001 Nov;6(1):115-21.

Prokopová I. Noradrenaline and behavior. *Cesk Fysiol.* 2010;59(2):51-8.

O'Donnell J et al. Norepinephrine: a neuromodulator that boosts the function of multiple cell types to optimize CNS performance. *Neurochem Res.* 2012 Nov;37(11):2496-512.

Zauner C et al. Resting energy expenditure in short-term starvation is increased as a result of an increase in serum norepinephrine. *The American Journal of Clinical Nutrition.* 2000 June;71(6):1511-1515.

Kurpad AV et al. Muscle and whole body metabolism after norepinephrine. *The American Journal of Physiology.* 1994 Jun;266(6 Pt 1):E877-84.

Nielsen T et al. Dissecting adipose tissue lipolysis: molecular regulation and implications for metabolic disease. *Journal of Molecular Endocrinology.* 2014 Jun;52(3):199-222.

SECTION FIVE

OpenStax, Anatomy & Physiology. 24.3 Lipid Metabolism. OpenStax CNX. Feb 26, 2016.

Browning JD et al. The effect of short-term fasting on liver and skeletal muscle lipid, glucose, and energy metabolism in healthy women and men. *J Lipid Res.* 2012 Mar;53(3):577-86.

Lei E et al. Fatty acids and their therapeutic potential in neurological disorders. *Neurochemistry International.* 2016 May;95:75-84.

Magistretti PJ, Allaman I. A cellular perspective on brain energy metabolism and functional imaging. *Neuron.* 2015 May 20;86(4):883-901.

Veech RL et al. Ketone bodies, potential therapeutic uses. *IUBMB Life.* 2001 Apr;51(4):241-7.

LaManna J.C. et al. (2009) Ketones Suppress Brain Glucose Consumption. In: Liss P., Hansell P., Bruley D.F., Harrison D.K. (eds)

Oxygen Transport to Tissue XXX. Advances in Experimental Medicine and Biology, vol 645. Springer, Boston, MA.

Lasse K et al. The glutamate/GABA-glutamine cycle: aspects of transport, neurotransmitter homeostasis and ammonia transfer. *Journal of Neurochemistry*. 2006 Jun;98(3):641-653.

Newsholm EA, Leech AR. Biochemistry for the medical sciences. Chichester, United Kingdom: John Wiley & Sons Ltd, 1983.

Greco T et al. Ketogenic diet decreases oxidative stress and improves mitochondrial respiratory complex activity. *J Cereb Blood Flow Metab*. 2016 Sep;36(9):1603-13.

Veech R et al. Ketone bodies mimic the life span extending properties of caloric restriction. *IUBMB Life*. 2017 May;69(5):305-314.

Maalouf M et al. Ketones inhibit mitochondrial production of reactive oxygen species production following glutamate excitotoxicity by increasing NADH oxidation. *Neuroscience*. 2007 Mar 2;145(1):256-64.

Phaniendra A et al. Free radicals: properties, sources, targets, and their implication in various diseases. *Indian J Clin Biochem*. 2015 Jan;30(1):11-26.

Rahal A et al. Oxidative Stress, Prooxidants, and Antioxidants: The Interplay. *BioMed Research International*. 2014:761264;19.

Hampton M et al. Inside the Neutrophil Phagosome: Oxidants, Myeloperoxidase, and Bacterial Killing. *Blood*. 1998 92:3007-3017.

Lobo V et al. Free radicals, antioxidants and functional foods: Impact on human health. *Pharmacogn Rev*. 2010 Jul-Dec;4(8):118-26.

Dizdaroglu M et al. Free radical-induced damage to DNA: mechanisms and measurement. *Free Radical Biology & Medicine*. 2002 Jun 1;32(11):1102-15.

Agarwal A et al. The role of free radicals and antioxidants in reproduction. *Current Opinion in Obstetrics and Gynecology*. 2006 Jun;18(3):325-32.

Huang WJ et al. Role of oxidative stress in Alzheimer's disease. *Biomed Rep.* 2016 May;4(5):519-522.

Miller ER 3rd et al. Meta-analysis: high-dosage vitamin E supplementation may increase all-cause mortality. *Ann Intern Med.* 2005 Jan 4;142(1):37-46.

Bjelakovic G et al. Antioxidant supplements for prevention of gastrointestinal cancers: a systematic review and meta-analysis. *The Lancet.* 2004 Oct 2-8;364(9441):1219-28.

Ristow M et al. Antioxidants prevent health-promoting effects of physical exercise in humans. *Proc Natl Acad Sci U S A.* 2009 May 26;106(21):8665-70.

Reger MA et al. Effects of beta-hydroxybutyrate on cognition in memory-impaired adults. *Neurobiology of Aging.* 2004 Mar;25(3):311-4.

SECTION SIX

Glick D et al. Autophagy: cellular and molecular mechanisms. *J Pathol.* 2010 May;221(1):3-12.

Mizushima N. Autophagy: process and function. *Genes & Dev.* 2007. 21: 2861-2873.

Bagherniya M et al. The effect of fasting or calorie restriction on autophagy induction: A review of the literature. *Ageing Research Reviews.* 2018 Nov;47:183-197.

He C et al. Exercise induces autophagy in peripheral tissues and in the brain. *Autophagy.* 2012;8(10):1548–1551.

Levine B, Klionsky DJ. Autophagy wins the 2016 Nobel Prize in Physiology or Medicine: Breakthroughs in baker's yeast fuel advances in biomedical research. *Proc Natl Acad Sci U S A.* 2017 Jan 10;114(2):201-205.

Alirezaei M et al. Short-term fasting induces profound neuronal autophagy. *Autophagy.* 2010 Aug 16;6(6):702-10.

Son JH et al. Neuronal autophagy and neurodegenerative diseases.

Exp Mol Med. 2012 Feb 29;44(2):89-98.

Zhang J et al. Intermittent Fasting Protects against Alzheimer's Disease Possible through Restoring Aquaporin-4 Polarity. *Front Mol Neurosci.* 2017 Nov 29;10:395.

Lynch-Day MA. The role of autophagy in Parkinson's disease. *Cold Spring Harb Perspect Med.* 2012 Apr;2(4):a009357.

Dagmar E et al. Preventing mutant huntingtin proteolysis and intermittent fasting promote autophagy in models of Huntington disease. *Acta Neuropathologica Communications - Neuroscience of Disease.* 2018 6:16.

Cheng CW et al. Prolonged fasting reduces IGF-1/PKA to promote hematopoietic-stem-cell-based regeneration and reverse immunosuppression. *Cell Stem Cell.* 2014 Jun 5;14(6):810-23.

Brandhorst S et al. A Periodic Diet that Mimics Fasting Promotes Multi-System Regeneration, Enhanced Cognitive Performance, and Healthspan. *Cell Metab.* 2015 Jul 7;22(1):86-99.

Devesa J et al. Multiple Effects of Growth Hormone in the Body: Is it Really the Hormone for Growth? *Clin Med Insights Endocrinol Diabetes.* 2016 Oct 12;9:47-71.

University Of Illinois At Chicago. Growth Hormone Activates Gene Involved In Healing Damaged Tissue. *ScienceDaily.* 4 December 2003.

Zhang Y et al. Ghrelin, growth hormone, and hepatic autophagy. *Proceedings of the National Academy of Sciences.* 2015 Jan;112 (4):1226-1231.

SECTION EIGHT

Braam B et al. Understanding the Two Faces of Low-Salt Intake. *Current Hypertension Reports.* 2017 Jun;19(6):49.

Katz DL. The Sodium Debate: More or Less About More or Less. *Integr Med (Encinitas).* 2014 Oct;13(5):29-31.

Rondon H, Badireddy M. Hyponatremia. [Updated 2018 Dec 13]. In: StatPearls [Internet]. Treasure Island (FL): StatPearls Publishing; 2019 Jan-. Available from: https://www.ncbi.nlm.nih.gov/books/NBK470386/

Weinsier R. Fasting—A review with emphasis on the electrolytes. *The American Journal Of Medicine.* 1971 Feb;50(2):223-240.

National Research Council (US) Committee on Diet and Health. Diet and Health: Implications for Reducing Chronic Disease Risk. Washington (DC): National Academies Press (US); 1989. 15, Electrolytes. Available from: https://www.ncbi.nlm.nih.gov/books/NBK218740/

National Research Council (US) Subcommittee on the Tenth Edition of the Recommended Dietary Allowances. Recommended Dietary Allowances: 10th Edition. Washington (DC): National Academies Press (US); 1989. 11, Water and Electrolytes. Available from: https://www.ncbi.nlm.nih.gov/books/NBK234935/

Runcie J. Urinary sodium and potassium excretion in fasting obese subjects. *Br Med J.* 1971;2(5752):22–25.

Funes SC et al. Effect of fasting in the digestive system: histological study of the small intestine in house sparrows. *Tissue & Cell.* 2014 Oct;46(5):356-62.

Schnitker MA et al. A clinical study of malnutrition in Japanese prisoners of war. *Annals of Internal Medicine.* 1951 Jul;35(1):69-96.

Mehanna H et al. Refeeding syndrome--awareness, prevention and management. *Head Neck Oncol.* 2009;1:4.

Part Five
Fasting and the Brain

SECTION ONE

Apple D et al. The role of adult neurogenesis in psychiatric and cognitive disorders. *Brain Research.* 2017 Jan;1655:270-276.

Cramer SC et al. Harnessing neuroplasticity for clinical applications. *Brain.* 2011;134(Pt 6):1591–1609.

Cattaneo A et al. The human BDNF gene: peripheral gene expression and protein levels as biomarkers for psychiatric disorders. *Transl Psychiatry.* 2016;6(11):e958.

Griffin ÉW et al. Aerobic exercise improves hippocampal function and increases BDNF in the serum of young adult males. *Physiology & Behaviour.* 2011 Oct 24;104(5):934-41.

Molendijk ML et al. Serum BDNF concentrations show strong seasonal variation and correlations with the amount of ambient sunlight. *PLoS One.* 2012;7(11):e48046.

Zielinski MR et al. Chronic sleep restriction elevates brain interleukin-1 beta and tumor necrosis factor-alpha and attenuates brain-derived neurotrophic factor expression. *Neurosci Lett.* 2014;580:27–31.

Rothman SM et al. Brain-derived neurotrophic factor as a regulator of systemic and brain energy metabolism and cardiovascular health. *Ann N Y Acad Sci.* 2012;1264(1):49–63.

Li L et al. Chronic intermittent fasting improves cognitive functions and brain structures in mice. *PLoS One.* 2013;8(6):e66069.

Mattson M et al. Beneficial effects of intermittent fasting and caloric restriction on the cardiovascular and cerebrovascular systems. *J Nutr Biochem.* 2005 Mar;16(3):129-37.

Sleiman SF et al. Exercise promotes the expression of brain derived neurotrophic factor (BDNF) through the action of the ketone body

B-hydroxybutyrate. *Elife*. 2016;5:e15092.

Maalouf M et al. The neuroprotective properties of calorie restriction, the ketogenic diet, and ketone bodies. *Brain Res Rev*. 2009;59(2):293–315.

Walsh J et al. Fasting and exercise differentially regulate BDNF mRNA expression in human skeletal muscle. *Applied Physiology Nutrition and Metabolism*. 2014 Sep;40(1):1-3.

Bastani A et al. The Effects of Fasting During Ramadan on the Concentration of Serotonin, Dopamine, Brain-Derived Neurotrophic Factor and Nerve Growth Factor. *Neurol Int*. 2017;9(2):7043.

Mattson MP et al. Meal size and frequency affect neuronal plasticity and vulnerability to disease: cellular and molecular mechanisms. *J Neurochem*. 2003 Feb;84(3):417-31.

Kowiański P et al. BDNF: A Key Factor with Multipotent Impact on Brain Signaling and Synaptic Plasticity. *Cell Mol Neurobiol*. 2018;38(3):579–593.

SECTION TWO

Rios M et al. Conditional deletion of brain-derived neurotrophic factor in the postnatal brain leads to obesity and hyperactivity. *Mol Endocrinol*. 2001 Oct;15(10):1748-57.

Lebrun B et al. Brain-derived neurotrophic factor (BDNF) and food intake regulation: a minireview. *Auton Neurosci*. 2006 Jun 30;126-127:30-8.

Gray J et al. Hyperphagia, severe obesity, impaired cognitive function, and hyperactivity associated with functional loss of one copy of the brain-derived neurotrophic factor (BDNF) gene. *Diabetes*. 2006;55(12):3366–3371.

Li B et al. Serum Levels of Brain-Derived Neurotrophic Factor Are Associated with Diabetes Risk, Complications, and Obesity: a Cohort

Study from Chinese Patients with Type 2 Diabetes. *Mol Neurobiol.* 2016 Oct;53(8):5492-9.

Krabbe, K.S et al. Brain-derived neurotrophic factor (BDNF) and type 2 diabetes. *Diabetologia.* 2007;50: 431.

Briana DD et al. Developmental origins of adult health and disease: The metabolic role of BDNF from early life to adulthood. *Metabolism.* 2018 Apr;81:45-51.

Pedersen BK et al. Role of exercise-induced brain-derived neurotrophic factor production in the regulation of energy homeostasis in mammals. *Experimental Physiology.* 2009 Dec;94(12):1153-60.

Pelleymounter MA et al. Characteristics of BDNF-induced weight loss. *Experimental Neurology.* 1995 Feb;131(2):229-38.

Shahid Z, Singh G. Physiology, Hypothalamus. [Updated 2018 Dec 9]. In: StatPearls [Internet]. Treasure Island (FL): StatPearls Publishing; 2019 Jan-. Available from: https://www.ncbi.nlm.nih.gov/books/NBK535380/

Unger TJ et al. Selective deletion of Bdnf in the ventromedial and dorsomedial hypothalamus of adult mice results in hyperphagic behavior and obesity. *J Neurosci.* 2007 Dec 26;27(52):14265-74.

Wang C et al. Brain-derived neurotrophic factor (BDNF) in the hypothalamic ventromedial nucleus increases energy expenditure. *Brain Res.* 2010;1336:66–77.

Tsuchida A et al. Acute effects of brain-derived neurotrophic factor on energy expenditure in obese diabetic mice. *Int J Obes Relat Metab Disord.* 2001 Sep;25(9):1286-93.

Nonomura T et al. Brain-derived neurotrophic factor regulates energy expenditure through the central nervous system in obese diabetic mice. *Int J Exp Diabetes Res.* 2001;2(3):201–209.

Velloso LA, Schwartz MW. Altered hypothalamic function in diet-induced obesity. *Int J Obes (Lond)*. 2011;35(12):1455–1465.

van de Sande-Lee S et al. [Hypothalamic dysfunction in obesity]. *Arq Bras Endocrinol Metabol*. 2012 Aug;56(6):341-50.

Mainardi M et al. Environment, Leptin Sensitivity, and Hypothalamic Plasticity. *Neural Plasticity*. 2013;438072.

Marosi K, Mattson MP. BDNF mediates adaptive brain and body responses to energetic challenges. *Trends Endocrinol Metab*. 2014;25(2):89–98.

Rosas-Vargas H et al. Brain-derived neurotrophic factor, food intake regulation, and obesity. *Archives of Medical Research*. 2011 Aug;42(6):482-94.

Berrettini W. The genetics of eating disorders. *Psychiatry (Edgmont)*. 2004;1(3):18–25.

Erickson KI et al. The aging hippocampus: interactions between exercise, depression, and BDNF. *Neuroscientist*. 2012;18(1):82–97.

SECTION THREE

Maguire EA, Gadian DG, Johnsrude IS, et al. Navigation-related structural change in the hippocampi of taxi drivers. *Proc Natl Acad Sci U S A*. 2000;97(8):4398–4403.

Duff MC et al. Hippocampal amnesia disrupts creative thinking. *Hippocampus*. 2013;23(12):1143–1149.

Beadle JN et al. Empathy in hippocampal amnesia. *Front Psychol*. 2013;4:69.

Rubin RD et al. The role of the hippocampus in flexible cognition and social behavior. *Front Hum Neurosci*. 2014;8:742.

SECTION FOUR

Lu B et al. BDNF and synaptic plasticity, cognitive function, and dysfunction. *Handbook of Experimental Pharmacology*.2014;220:223-50.

McGinty JF et al. Brain-derived neurotrophic factor and cocaine addiction. *Brain Res.* 2009;1314:183–193.

Pandey SC et al. Central and medial amygdaloid brain-derived neurotrophic factor signaling plays a critical role in alcohol-drinking and anxiety-like behaviors. *The Journal of Neuroscience.* 2006 Aug 9;26(32):8320-31.

Berglind WJ et al. A BDNF infusion into the medial prefrontal cortex suppresses cocaine seeking in rats. *The European Journal of Neuroscience.* 2007 Aug;26(3):757-66.

Zanardini R et al. Alterations of brain-derived neurotrophic factor serum levels in patients with alcohol dependence. *Alcoholism, Clinical and Experimental Research.* 2011 Aug;35(8):1529-33.

Gordon EL et al. What Is the Evidence for "Food Addiction?" A Systematic Review. *Nutrients.* 2018;10(4):477.

van Strien T. Causes of Emotional Eating and Matched Treatment of Obesity. *Curr Diab Rep.* 2018;18(6):35.

Duckworth AL. The significance of self-control. *Proc Natl Acad Sci U S A.* 2011;108(7):2639–2640.

Verma D et al. Hunger Promotes Fear Extinction by Activation of an Amygdala Microcircuit. *Neuropsychopharmacology.* 2016;41(2):431–439.

LeDoux JE. Emotion circuits in the brain. *Annu Rev Neurosci.* 2000;23:155-84.

Mobbs D et al. When fear is near: threat imminence elicits prefrontal-periaqueductal gray shifts in humans. *Science.* 2007;317(5841):1079–1083.

Shi L et al. Fasting enhances extinction retention and prevents the return of fear in humans. *Translational Psychiatry.* 2018;8(214)

Shin LM, Liberzon I. The neurocircuitry of fear, stress, and anxiety disorders. *Neuropsychopharmacology.* 2010;35(1):169–191.

SECTION FIVE

NHS digital. Prescriptions Dispensed in the Community - Statistics for England, 2006-2016. 29 Jun 2017.

Mojtabai R. Increase in Antidepressant Medication in the US Adult Population between 1990 and 2003. *Psychother Psychosom*. 2008;77:83–92.

Lépine JP, Briley M. The increasing burden of depression. *Neuropsychiatr Dis Treat*. 2011;7(Suppl 1):3–7.

Baj G et al. Physical exercise and antidepressants enhance BDNF targeting in hippocampal CA3 dendrites: further evidence of a spatial code for BDNF splice variants. *Neuropsychopharmacology*. 2012;37(7):1600-11.

Mulder RT. An epidemic of depression or the medicalization of distress? *Perspectives in Biology and Medicine*. 2008 Spring;51(2):238-50.

Mental Health & Suicide Prevention. WHO 2019

Siuciak J et al. Antidepressant-Like Effect of Brain-derived Neurotrophic Factor (BDNF). *Pharmacology Biochemistry and Behavior*. 1997 Jan;56(1):131-137.

Hashimoto K. Brain-derived neurotrophic factor as a biomarker for mood disorders: an historical overview and future directions. *Psychiatry and Clinical Neurosciences*. 2010 Aug;64(4):341-57.

Celik Guzel E et al. Can low brain-derived neurotrophic factor levels be a marker of the presence of depression in obese women? *Neuropsychiatr Dis Treat*. 2014;10:2079-86.

Cattaneo A et al. The human BDNF gene: peripheral gene expression and protein levels as biomarkers for psychiatric disorders. *Transl Psychiatry*. 2016;6(11):e958.

Dwivedi Y. Brain-derived neurotrophic factor: role in depression and suicide. *Neuropsychiatr Dis Treat*. 2009;5:433–449.

Blouin AM et al. Human hypocretin and melanin-concentrating hormone levels are linked to emotion and social interaction. *Nat Commun.* 2013;4:1547.

SECTION SIX

Hasenkamp W. Using First-Person Reports During Meditation to Investigate Basic Cognitive Experience. *Meditation – Neuroscientific Approaches and Philosophical Implications.* 2013 Oct;75-93.

Seeley WW et al. Dissociable intrinsic connectivity networks for salience processing and executive control. *J Neurosci.* 2007;27(9):2349–2356.

Carhart-Harris RL, Friston KJ. The default-mode, ego-functions and free-energy: a neurobiological account of Freudian ideas. *Brain.* 2010;133(Pt 4):1265–1283.

Carhart-Harris RL et al. Neural correlates of the psychedelic state as determined by fMRI studies with psilocybin. *Proceedings of the National Academy of Sciences.* 2012 Feb;109(6):2138-2143.

Mak L et al. The Default Mode Network in Healthy Individuals: A Systematic Review and Meta-Analysis. *Brain Connectivity.* 2017 Feb;7(1).

Buckner RL et al. The brain's default network: anatomy, function, and relevance to disease. *Annals of the New York Academy of Sciences.* 2008 Mar;1124:1-38.

Hasenkamp W et al. Mind wandering and attention during focused meditation: a fine-grained temporal analysis of fluctuating cognitive states. *Neuroimage.* 2012 Jan 2;59(1):750-60.

Garrison KA et al. Meditation leads to reduced default mode network activity beyond an active task. *Cogn Affect Behav Neurosci.* 2015 Sep;15(3):712-20.

Brewer JA et al. Meditation experience is associated with differences in default mode network activity and connectivity. *Proc Natl Acad Sci U*

S A. 2011 Dec 13;108(50):20254-9.

Šimleša M et al. The Flow Engine Framework: A Cognitive Model of Optimal Human Experience. *Eur J Psychol*. 2018;14(1):232–253.

Harris D et al. Chapter 12 - Neurocognitive mechanisms of the flow state. *Progress in Brain Research*. 2017;234:221-243.

Orfanos S et al. Investigating the impact of overnight fasting on intrinsic functional connectivity: a double-blind fMRI study. *Brain Imaging Behav*. 2018;12(4):1150-1159.

SECTION SEVEN

Wheless JW. History of the ketogenic diet. *Epilepsia*. 2008 Nov;49 Suppl 8:3-5.

Shorvon S. Drug treatment of epilepsy in the century of the ILAE: The first 50 years, 1909–1958. *Epilepsia*. 2009 Mar:50(3):69-92.

Hartman AL et al. The neuropharmacology of the ketogenic diet. *Pediatr Neurol*. 2007;36(5):281–292.

McNally MA, Hartman AL. Ketone bodies in epilepsy. *J Neurochem*. 2012;121(1):28–35.

Barañano KW, Hartman AL. The ketogenic diet: uses in epilepsy and other neurologic illnesses. *Curr Treat Options Neurol*. 2008;10(6):410–419.

Kashiwaya Y et al. D-beta-hydroxybutyrate protects neurons in models of Alzheimer's and Parkinson's disease. *Proc Natl Acad Sci U S A*. 2000;97(10):5440–5444.

Lei E et al. Fatty acids and their therapeutic potential in neurological disorders. *Neurochemistry International*. 2016 May;95:75-84.

Cobley JN et al. 13 reasons why the brain is susceptible to oxidative stress. *Redox Biol*. 2018;15:490–503.

Song P, Zou MH. Roles of reactive oxygen species in physiology and pathology. *Atherosclerosis: risks, mechanisms, and therapies* (Wang H,

Patterson C, eds), pp 379-392.

Gandhi S, Abramov A. Mechanism of Oxidative Stress in Neurodegeneration. *Oxidative Medicine and Cellular Longevity.* 2012;428010.

Federico A et al. Mitochondria, oxidative stress and neurodegeneration. *J Neurol Sci.* 2012 Nov 15;322(1-2):254-62.

Patten DA et al. Reactive oxygen species: stuck in the middle of neurodegeneration. *J Alzheimers Dis.* 2010;20 Suppl 2:S357-67.

Wang X et al. Oxidative stress and mitochondrial dysfunction in Alzheimer's disease. *Biochim Biophys Acta.* 2014;1842(8):1240–1247.

Zhao Y, Zhao B. Oxidative stress and the pathogenesis of Alzheimer's disease. *Oxid Med Cell Longev.* 2013;2013:316523.

Chen L et al. Lipid peroxidation up-regulates BACE1 expression in vivo: a possible early event of amyloidogenesis in Alzheimer's disease. *J Neurochem.* 2008;107(1):197–207.

Blesa J et al. Oxidative stress and Parkinson's disease. *Front Neuroanat.* 2015;9:91.

Schapira AH. Mitochondria in the aetiology and pathogenesis of Parkinson's disease. *Lancet Neurol.* 2008 Jan;7(1):97-109.

Uttara B et al. Oxidative stress and neurodegenerative diseases: a review of upstream and downstream antioxidant therapeutic options. *Curr Neuropharmacol.* 2009;7(1):65–74.

Huang WJ et al. Role of oxidative stress in Alzheimer's disease. *Biomed Rep.* 2016;4(5):519–522.

Moosmann B, Behl C. Antioxidants as treatment for neurodegenerative disorders. *Expert Opin Investig Drugs.* 2002 Oct;11(10):1407-35.

Murphy MP. Antioxidants as therapies: can we improve on nature? *Free Radic Biol Med.* 2014 Jan;66:20-3.

Kohen R. Skin antioxidants: their role in aging and in oxidative stress--new approaches for their evaluation. *Biomed Pharmacother.* 1999 May;53(4):181-92.

Rudman D et al. Effects of human growth hormone in men over 60 years old. *The New England Journal of Medicine.* 1990 Jul 5;323(1):1-6.

Reed ML et al. Adult growth hormone deficiency - benefits, side effects, and risks of growth hormone replacement. *Front Endocrinol (Lausanne).* 2013;4:64.

McGregor RA et al. It is not just muscle mass: a review of muscle quality, composition and metabolism during ageing as determinants of muscle function and mobility in later life. *Longev Healthspan.* 2014;3(1):9.

McLeod M et al. Live strong and prosper: the importance of skeletal muscle strength for healthy ageing. *Biogerontology.* 2016;17(3):497–510.

Magon N et al. Growth hormone in the management of female infertility. *Indian J Endocrinol Metab.* 2011;15 Suppl 3(Suppl3):S246–S247.

Galdiero M et al. Growth hormone, prolactin, and sexuality. 2012 Sep;35(8):782-94.

Becker AJ et al. Serum levels of human growth hormone during different penile conditions in the cavernous and systemic blood of healthy men and patients with erectile dysfunction. *Urology.* 2002 Apr;59(4):609-14.

Part Six
Fasting for the Future

SECTION ONE

Tuso P. Prediabetes and lifestyle modification: time to prevent a preventable disease. *Perm J.* 2014;18(3):88–93.

Tabák AG et al. Prediabetes: a high-risk state for diabetes development. *Lancet.* 2012;379(9833):2279–2290.

Sutton E et al. Early Time-Restricted Feeding Improves Insulin Sensitivity, Blood Pressure, and Oxidative Stress Even without Weight Loss in Men with Prediabetes. *Cell Metabolism.* 2018 Jun:27(6):1212-1221.

Max Roser and Esteban Ortiz-Ospina (2019) - "Global Extreme Poverty". Published online at OurWorldInData.org. Retrieved from: 'https://ourworldindata.org/extreme-poverty'

Max Roser (2019) - "Life Expectancy". Published online at OurWorldInData.org. Retrieved from: 'https://ourworldindata.org/life-expectancy'

American Diabetes Association. Economic costs of diabetes in the U.S. in 2012. *Diabetes Care.* 2013;36(4):1033–1046.

Huang E et al. Projecting the Future Diabetes Population Size and Related Costs for the U.S. *Diabetes Care.* 2009 Dec; 32(12): 2225-2229.

Diabetes Statistics. 30 October 2018. World Health Organization.

Elliot RB. Diabetes--a man made disease. *Medical Hypotheses.* 2006;67(2):388-91.

Furmli S et al. Therapeutic use of intermittent fasting for people with type 2 diabetes as an alternative to insulin. *Case Reports.* 2018;2018:bcr 2017-221854.

Arnason TG et al. Effects of intermittent fasting on health markers in those with type 2 diabetes: A pilot study. *World J Diabetes.* 2017;8(4):154–164.

Grajower MM, Horne BD. Clinical Management of Intermittent Fasting in Patients with Diabetes Mellitus. *Nutrients*. 2019 Apr 18;11(4).

SECTION TWO

Myers MG Jr et al. Obesity and leptin resistance: distinguishing cause from effect. *Trends Endocrinol Metab*. 2010;21(11):643–651.

Crujeiras AB et al. Weight regain after a diet-induced loss is predicted by higher baseline leptin and lower ghrelin plasma levels. *J Clin Endocrinol Metab*. 2010 Nov;95(11):5037-44.

SECTION THREE

Friedrich M. Global Obesity Epidemic Worsening. *JAMA*. 2017;318(7):603.

Cawley J, Meyerhoefer C. The medical care costs of obesity: an instrumental variables approach. *Journal of Health Economics*. 2012 Jan;31(1):219-30.

Public Health England. Health matters: obesity and the food environment. Published 31 March 2017.

Wang YC et al. Health and economic burden of the projected obesity trends in the USA and the UK. *Lancet*. 2011 Aug 27;378(9793):815-25.

Djalalinia S et al. Health impacts of Obesity. *Pak J Med Sci*. 2015;31(1):239–242.

Pi-Sunyer X. The medical risks of obesity. *Postgrad Med*. 2009;121(6):21–33.

Luppino FS et al. Overweight, obesity, and depression: a systematic review and meta-analysis of longitudinal studies. *Arch Gen Psychiatry*. 2010 Mar;67(3):220-9.

DiNicolantonio JJ et al. Lorcaserin for the treatment of obesity? A closer look at its side effects. *Open Heart*. 2014;1:e000173.

SECTION FOUR

Galgani J, Ravussin E. Energy metabolism, fuel selection and body weight regulation. *Int J Obes (Lond)*. 2008;32 Suppl 7(Suppl 7):S109–S119.

Ibrahim MM. Subcutaneous and visceral adipose tissue: structural and functional differences. *Obesity Reviews: an official journal of the International Association for the Study of Obesity*. 2010 Jan;11(1):11-8.

Porter SA et al. Abdominal subcutaneous adipose tissue: a protective fat depot? *Diabetes Care*. 2009;32(6):1068–1075.

Koh-Banerjee P et al. Changes in body weight and body fat distribution as risk factors for clinical diabetes in US men. *American Journal of Epidemiology*. 2004 Jun 15;159(12):1150-9.

Pascot A et al. Age-related increase in visceral adipose tissue and body fat and the metabolic risk profile of premenopausal women. *Diabetes Care*. 1999 Sep;22(9):1471-8.

Walker SP et al. Body size and fat distribution as predictors of stroke among US men. *American Journal of Epidemiology*. 1996 Dec 15;144(12):1143-50.

Nicklas BJ et al. Abdominal obesity is an independent risk factor for chronic heart failure in older people. *Journal of the American Geriatrics Society*. 2006 Mar;54(3):413-20.

Whitmer RA et al. Central obesity and increased risk of dementia more than three decades later. *Neurology*. 2008 Sep 30;71(14):1057-64.

Razay G et al. Obesity, abdominal obesity and Alzheimer disease. *Dementia and Geriatric Cognitive Disorders*. 2006;22(2):173-6.

'Taking aim at belly fat.' Harvard Health Publishing August 2010.

Ding H et al. Fasting induces a subcutaneous-to-visceral fat switch mediated by microRNA-149-3p and suppression of PRDM16. *Nat Commun*. 2016;7:11533.

Tang HN et al. Plasticity of adipose tissue in response to fasting and refeeding in male mice. *Nutr Metab (Lond)*. 2017;14:3.

Gjedsted J et al. Effects of a 3-day fast on regional lipid and glucose metabolism in human skeletal muscle and adipose tissue. *Acta Physiologica (Oxford, England)*. 2007 Nov;191(3):205-16.

Johannsson G et al. Growth hormone treatment of abdominally obese men reduces abdominal fat mass, improves glucose and lipoprotein metabolism, and reduces diastolic blood pressure. *The Journal of Clinical Endocrinology and Metabolism*. 1997 Mar;82(3):727-34.

Bengtsson BA et al. Treatment of adults with growth hormone (GH) deficiency with recombinant human GH. *The Journal of Clinical Endocrinology and Metabolism*. 1993 Feb;76(2):309-17.

Taaffe DR et al. Recombinant human growth hormone, but not insulin-like growth factor-I, enhances central fat loss in postmenopausal women undergoing a diet and exercise program. *Hormone and Metabolic Research*. 2001 Mar;33(3):156-62.

Miller K et al. Truncal Adiposity, Relative Growth Hormone Deficiency, and Cardiovascular Risk. *The Journal of Clinical Endocrinology & Metabolism*. 2005 Feb;90(2):768-774.

Ottosson M et al. Effects of cortisol and growth hormone on lipolysis in human adipose tissue. *The Journal of Clinical Endocrinology and Metabolism*. 2000 Feb;85(2):799-803.

Stanley TL, Grinspoon SK. Effects of growth hormone-releasing hormone on visceral fat, metabolic, and cardiovascular indices in human studies. *Growth Horm IGF Res*. 2014;25(2):59–65.

Beauregard C et al. Growth hormone decreases visceral fat and improves cardiovascular risk markers in women with hypopituitarism: a randomized, placebo-controlled study. *J Clin Endocrinol Metab*. 2008;93(6):2063–2071.

Sakharova AA et al. Role of growth hormone in regulating lipolysis, proteolysis, and hepatic glucose production during fasting. *J Clin Endocrinol Metab.* 2008;93(7):2755–2759.

SECTION FIVE

Qi L, Cho YA. Gene-environment interaction and obesity. *Nutr Rev.* 2008;66(12):684–694.

Hallal PC et al. Global physical activity levels: surveillance progress, pitfalls, and prospects. *Lancet.* 2012 Jul 21;380(9838):247-57.

Schoeller DA, Jefford G. Determinants of the energy costs of light activities: inferences for interpreting doubly labeled water data. *International Journal of Obesity and Related Metabolic Disorders.* 2002 Jan;26(1):97-101.

Castellani W et al. Adherence to structured physical exercise in overweight and obese subjects: a review of psychological models. *Eat Weight Disord.* 2003 Mar;8(1):1-11.

Ekblom-Bak E et al. The importance of non-exercise physical activity for cardiovascular health and longevity. *Br J Sports Med.* 2014 Feb;48(3):233-8.

Katzmarzyk PT et al. Sitting time and mortality from all causes, cardiovascular disease, and cancer. *Med Sci Sports Exerc.* 2009 May;41(5):998-1005.

Manini TM et al. Modifying effect of obesity on the association between sitting and incident diabetes in post-menopausal women. *Obesity (Silver Spring).* 2014;22(4):1133–1141.

Villablanca PA et al. Nonexercise activity thermogenesis in obesity management. *Mayo Clinic Proceedings.* 2015 Apr;90(4):509-19.

Kraybill D (September 27, 2001). The Riddle of Amish Culture (Revised ed.). Johns Hopkins University Press. ISBN 978-0801867729.

Bassett DR et al. Physical activity in an Old Order Amish community. *Med Sci Sports Exerc.* 2004 Jan;36(1):79-85.

Bassett DR et al. Pedometer-measured physical activity and health behaviors in U.S. adults. *Med Sci Sports Exerc.* 2010;42(10):1819–1825.

Levine JA et al. Interindividual variation in posture allocation: possible role in human obesity. *Science.* 2005 Jan 28;307(5709):584-6.

Kiwaki K et al. Orexin A (hypocretin 1) injected into the hypothalamic paraventricular nucleus and spontaneous physical activity in rats. *Am J Physiol Endocrinol Metab.* 2004 Apr;286(4):E551-9.

Hara J et al. Genetic ablation of orexin neurons in mice results in narcolepsy, hypophagia, and obesity. *Neuron.* 2001 May;30(2):345-54.

John J et al. Systemic administration of hypocretin-1 reduces cataplexy and normalizes sleep and waking durations in narcoleptic dogs. *Sleep Res Online.* 2000;3(1):23-8.

Nixon JP et al. Sleep disorders, obesity, and aging: the role of orexin. *Ageing Res Rev.* 2015;20:63–73.

SECTION SIX

Jastreboff AM et al. Neural correlates of stress- and food cue-induced food craving in obesity: association with insulin levels. *Diabetes Care.* 2013;36(2):394–402.

Tryon MS et al. Having your cake and eating it too: a habit of comfort food may link chronic social stress exposure and acute stress-induced cortisol hyporesponsiveness. *Physiol Behav.* 2013 Apr 10;114-115:32-7.

Abizaid A. Stress and obesity: The ghrelin connection. *J Neuroendocrinol.* 2019 Feb 3:e12693.

Adam TC, Epel ES. Stress, eating and the reward system. *Physiol Behav.* 2007 Jul 24;91(4):449-58.

Buss J et al. Associations of ghrelin with eating behaviors, stress, metabolic factors, and telomere length among overweight and obese women: preliminary evidence of attenuated ghrelin effects in obesity? *Appetite.* 2014;76:84–94.

Tomiyama AJ et al. Comfort food is comforting to those most stressed: evidence of the chronic stress response network in high stress women. Psychoneuroendocrinology. 2011;36(10):1513–1519.

Xenaki N et al. Impact of a stress management program on weight loss, mental health and lifestyle in adults with obesity: a randomized controlled trial. *J Mol Biochem*. 2018;7(2):78–84.

World Health Organization. Obesity and overweight statistics. 16 February 2018.

SECTION SEVEN

Hunter P. The inflammation theory of disease. The growing realization that chronic inflammation is crucial in many diseases opens new avenues for treatment. *EMBO Rep*. 2012;13(11):968–970.

Lavin DN, Joesting JJ, Chiu GS, et al. Fasting induces an anti-inflammatory effect on the neuroimmune system which a high-fat diet prevents. *Obesity (Silver Spring)*. 2011;19(8):1586–1594.

Mattson MP, Longo VD, Harvie M. Impact of intermittent fasting on health and disease processes. *Ageing Res Rev*. 2017;39:46–58.

Hafström I et al. Effects of fasting on disease activity, neutrophil function, fatty acid composition, and leukotriene biosynthesis in patients with rheumatoid arthritis. *Arthritis Rheum*. 1988 May;31(5):585-92.

Clipped from Page 4 of the The Brooklyn Daily Eagle, Brooklyn, New York. 31 Dec 1918.

Youm Y et al. The ketone metabolite B-hydroxybutyrate blocks NLRP3 inflammasome–mediated inflammatory disease. *Nature Medicine*. 2015 Feb;21:263-269.

Doi Y et al. Relationship Between C-Reactive Protein and Glucose Levels in Community-Dwelling Subjects Without Diabetes. *Diabetes Care*. 2005 May;28(5):1211-1213.

Aronson D et al. Association between fasting glucose and C-reactive protein in middle-aged subjects. *Diabet Med.* 2004 Jan;21(1):39-44.

Sproston NR, Ashworth JJ. Role of C-Reactive Protein at Sites of Inflammation and Infection. *Front Immunol.* 2018;9:754.

Moro T et al. Effects of eight weeks of time-restricted feeding (16/8) on basal metabolism, maximal strength, body composition, inflammation, and cardiovascular risk factors in resistance-trained males. *Journal of Translational Medicine.* 2016 Oct;14(290).

Gil-Campos M et al. Adiponectin, the missing link in insulin resistance and obesity. *Clin Nutr.* 2004 Oct;23(5):963-74.

Chandran M et al. Adiponectin: More Than Just Another Fat Cell Hormone? *Diabetes Care.* 2003 Aug; 26(8): 2442-2450.

Yoon JM et al. Adiponectin Increases Fatty Acid Oxidation in Skeletal Muscle Cells by Sequential Activation of AMP-Activated Protein Kinase, p38 Mitogen-Activated Protein Kinase, and Peroxisome Proliferator–Activated Receptor. *Diabetes.* Sep 2006, 55 (9) 2562-2570.

Yamauchi T et al. Adiponectin stimulates glucose utilization and fatty-acid oxidation by activating AMP-activated protein kinase. *Nature Medicine.* 2002;8:1288-1295.

Al Maskari MY, Alnaqdy AA. Correlation between Serum Leptin Levels, Body Mass Index and Obesity in Omanis. *Sultan Qaboos Univ Med J.* 2006;6(2):27–31.

Matsubara M et al. Inverse relationship between plasma adiponectin and leptin concentrations in normal-weight and obese women. *Eur J Endocrinol.* 2002 Aug;147(2):173-80.

Yadav A et al. Role of leptin and adiponectin in insulin resistance. *Clin Chim Acta.* 2013 Feb 18;417:80-4.

Gulcelik NE et al. Adipocytokines and aging: adiponectin and leptin. *Minerva Endocrinol.* 2013 Jun;38(2):203-10.

Li S et al. Adiponectin levels and risk of type 2 diabetes: a systematic review and meta-analysis. *JAMA*. 2009 Jul 8;302(2):179-88.

Yokoyama H et al. Plasma Adiponectin Level Is Associated with Insulin-Stimulated Nonoxidative Glucose Disposal. *The Journal of Clinical Endocrinology & Metabolism*. 2006 Jan;91(1):290-294.

Ziemke F, Mantzoros CS. Adiponectin in insulin resistance: lessons from translational research. *Am J Clin Nutr*. 2010;91(1):258S–261S.

Ghantous CM et al. Differential Role of Leptin and Adiponectin in Cardiovascular System. *International Journal of Endocrinology*. 2015;534320.

Caselli C et al. Back to the heart: the protective role of adiponectin. *Pharmacol Res*. 2014 Apr;82:9-20.

Hui X et al. Adiponectin and cardiovascular health: an update. *Br J Pharmacol*. 2012;165(3):574–590.

Pi-Sunyer X. The medical risks of obesity. *Postgrad Med*. 2009;121(6):21–33.

Abdelaal M et al. Morbidity and mortality associated with obesity. *Ann Transl Med*. 2017;5(7):161.

SECTION EIGHT

Kasser T et al. Time Affluence as a Path toward Personal Happiness and Ethical Business Practice: Empirical Evidence from Four Studies. *Journal of Business Ethics*. 2009;84:243–255.

Roxburgh S. "There Just Aren't Enough Hours in the Day": The Mental Health Consequences of Time Pressure. *Journal of Health and Social Behavior*. 2004;45(2):115–131.

Banwell C et al. Reflections on expert consensus: a case study of the social trends contributing to obesity. *European Journal of Public Health*. 2005 Dec;15(6):564-568.

Escoto KH et al. Work hours and perceived time barriers to healthful eating among young adults. *Am J Health Behav*. 2012;36(6):786–796.

Part Seven
Feed the Positive, Starve the Negative

Goldhamer AC et al. Medically supervised water-only fasting in the treatment of borderline hypertension. *Journal of Alternative and Complementary Medicine*. 2002 Oct;8(5):643-50.

Beleslin B et al. The effects of three-week fasting diet on blood pressure, lipid profile and glucoregulation in extremely obese patients. *Srp Arh Celok Lek*. 2007 Jul-Aug;135(7-8):440-6.

Andersson B et al. Acute effects of short-term fasting on blood pressure, circulating noradrenaline and efferent sympathetic nerve activity. *Acta Medica Scandinavica*. 1988;223(6):485-90.

Lindsay M et al. 20.2 Blood Flow, Blood Pressure, and Resistance. *Anatomy & Physiology*. Chapter 20: The Cardiovascular System: Blood Vessels and Circulation.

Lee B et al. Standardization of penile blood flow parameters in normal men using intracavernous prostaglandin E1 and visual sexual stimulation. *The Journal of Urology*. 1993 Jan;149(1):49-52.

Azadzoi KM, Siroky MB. Neurologic factors in female sexual function and dysfunction. *Korean J Urol*. 2010;51(7):443–449.

Galdiero M et al. Growth hormone, prolactin, and sexuality. *Journal of Endocrinological Investigation*. 2012 Sep;35(8):782-94.

Becker AJ et al. Serum levels of human growth hormone during different penile conditions in the cavernous and systemic blood of healthy men and patients with erectile dysfunction. *Urology*. 2002 Apr;59(4):609-14.

Boutrel B et al. The role of hypocretin in driving arousal and goal-oriented behaviors. *Brain Res*. 2009;1314:103–111.

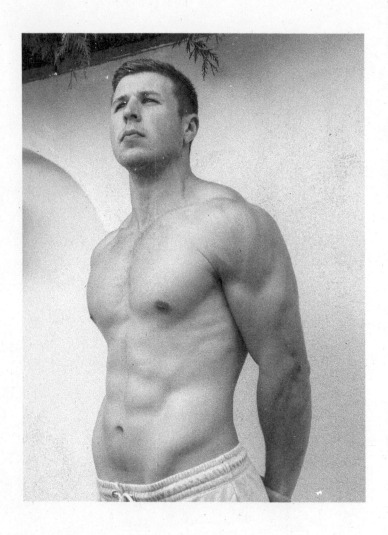

My name is Scott Murray.

And I don't have any letters after my name.

The discovery of fasting changed my life. Previously, I had a very unhealthy relationship with food and possibly even myself. I had allowed my pursuit of a 'healthy' lifestyle to take precedence over all else and subtract from the quality of my life and the lives of those close to me.

Incorporating fasting has given me freedom. But it has also sent me on a path of inquiry which encourages me to dig deeper and question everything. However, there is still a lack of information about it. And many people dismiss it as nonsense or a fad. Because of this, I felt compelled to write this book. It is a book I wish I could have read a few years ago. And I think it can transmit a lot of value for many people.

If you would like to know more about me, you can find me on the socials (I'm most active on Instagram and YouTube) under the name **goodlifetheory.**

www.goodlifetheory.com